MW01538195

Hospital

HOSPITAL COPY

BEDREST BEFORE BABY:

WHAT'S A MOTHER TO DO?

A SURVIVAL HANDBOOK FOR HIGH-RISK MOMS

BEDREST BEFORE BABY:

WHAT'S A MOTHER TO DO?

A SURVIVAL HANDBOOK FOR HIGH-RISK MOMS

By Patricia D. Isennock, R.N., M.S., "Mom"

BEDREST BEFORE BABY: WHAT'S A MOTHER TO DO?

A Survival Handbook for High-risk Moms

By Patricia D. Isennock, R.N., M.S.

Published by: Mustard Seed Publications

All rights reserved. No part of this book may be reproduced or transmitted in any form or by any means, electronic or mechanical, including photocopying, recording or by any information storage and retrieval system without written permission from the author, except for the inclusion of brief quotations in a review.

Copyright © 1992, 1995 by Patricia D. Isennock
  First Printing 1992
  Second Printing 1995, revised
  Printed in the United States of America

Library of Congress Cataloging in Publication Data
Isennock, Patricia D.
  BEDREST BEFORE BABY: WHAT'S A MOTHER TO DO?
  A Survival Handbook for High-risk Moms
  Library of Congress Catalog Card Number: 95-75282

ISBN 0-9632392-6-0 $12.95 Softcover

To Michael,
Matthew, Christopher, and Patrick
for all their love and support

ACKNOWLEDGMENTS

Many thanks are due to the large number of family, friends and colleagues who assisted and supported me in this project. My husband, Michael, has been my main source of encouragement. Mary Donohue, my Mom, has always been my greatest role model. My dad, John A. Donohue, always told me I could do anything with a little faith.

I am eternally grateful to the entire staff of Unit 26 at Greater Baltimore Medical Center. They not only cared for me through two months of hospitalized bedrest for pregnancy, they have contributed in numerous ways to the completion of the book.

This book is easier to read thanks to the diligent editorial work of Mary Donohue, Rebecca Drinks, Gina Robinson, R.N., Cheryl Giese, R.N., Joseph C. Donohue, Ph.D. and Christel Riley, R.N.

JodyLynn Kovalczyck, Gina Robinson, and Mary Anne Lewis stand out among the many mothers on bedrest who have added their personal experiences and suggestions.

Nancy Campbell and Debbie Jones have been a font of social services information.

The faithful visits of my pastors, Rev. Elmer J. Klein and Rev. Donald Beutel, sustained my hope during my hospitalization. It was Pastor Klein's request that I "write it down for others" which initiated this project.

Nancy Kay Leatherman enthusiastically provided invaluable computer assistance.

I also wish to thank Jan Bavis, Lisa Deickman, Kim Lindner, and Ann McClean for posing.

PHOTOS: Peggy Eifert

COVER: Jim Geckle and Jack Shipley

DISCLAIMER

This book is not intended to provide medical services. It is in no way intended to be a substitute for any medical or nursing care. Professional obstetrical services should be obtained by any woman who is, thinks she may be, or plans to be pregnant.

Every attempt has been made to verify that the information contained in this book is as current as the date of printing. The reader is advised to verify individual plans of care with her health care professional.

The author and the publisher of this book shall not be liable for any loss or damage resulting from the information contained herein.

BEDREST BEFORE BABY:
WHAT'S A MOTHER TO DO?

INTRODUCTION

Having a baby is supposed to be the most natural act in the world. It is a joyous occasion. People do it all the time! So ... how did you get into this predicament? Why can't you be enjoying this pregnancy vertically? Because you've joined thousands of other mothers-to-be who have been labelled "high risk." High risk pregnancy has a myriad of causes, experiences, and outcomes. Most often, it means being on bed rest at some time and in some fashion. This is no picnic! I know ... I've been there.

Michael and I tried to get pregnant for six years. We watched the calendar, checked basal body temperature, monitored mucous consistency, and acted at the appropriate times. Then Michael had semen studies (sperm analysis) while I underwent a hysterosalpingogram (an X-ray exam of the uterus and tubes). His sperm was plentiful and robust; my tubes were unobstructed. I did have a stenotic (tightly closed) cervix and an abnormally shaped uterus. Both of these conditions were attributed to DES exposure. My mom, after experiencing several miscarriages, had taken DES (Diethylstilbesterol) to maintain her pregnancy with me as well as with my two sisters and one brother. My cervix was so tight, it may not have allowed sperm to enter. Or the abnormal shape of my uterus may have caused fertilized eggs to abort very early. In either case, we faced surgery and hormones or adoption.

The next year we privately adopted our first son, Matthew. It was miraculous! We were legal guardians from birth and legal parents in six months. Within that time, I also became pregnant but it was an ectopic, or tubal pregnancy. Having a tube removed further decreased our chances of ever having a biological child. Two years later we spread the word that we would like to adopt again. Unsuccessfully, we contacted several agencies. Then we realized our second miracle ... I was pregnant again.

Christopher was born two months early and, thus, spent a month in a neonatal intensive care unit (NICU) and a year on an apnea monitor due to a digestive disorder. At this writing, he is a hale and hearty eight-year-old. His first year was a chaotic and sleepless one for us. Romantic moments were rare, but it took only one to produce our third miracle. Before Christopher was off the monitor I had another positive pregnancy test.

This time I took no chances. Immediately, I made an appointment with obstetricians who managed high risk pregnancies. Doctors Zern and Facciolo reassured me by their careful monitoring at biweekly office visits. By fourteen weeks, however, my cervix had begun to dilate. Five weeks later, it had progressed so that I required a cervical suture to keep it closed. It was at this time that my bed rest started. My doctors were very careful to explain to Michael and me that maintaining this pregnancy would require a commitment. The extent of that commitment would be revealed at 26 weeks when I started in premature labor.

I am a nurse. I was a nurse before we had any children. I had worked in hospitals, for the health department, in nursing education programs, and in outpatient clinics. My last pregnancy test was done while I was working in a high risk obstetrics clinic. Professionally, I knew what would be required, but I had just begun to discover what was involved personally.

Bed rest? You mean take it easy, no jogging. Total bed rest? You mean ... only get out of bed to go to the bathroom? ... on good days? But ... I have two little boys to take care of ... one is not even walking yet ... But I have to work to pay the bills ... and the bills - I don't know if my insurance will cover this ... How will Michael manage - he has to work, too ... and what about my brother's wedding ... What am I going to do?!

That is when this book started. We managed to survive, though not without a few struggles. And Patrick William is our daily joyful reminder.

Although we had survived an abnormal pregnancy, the bills had not disappeared. I soon found myself working on the same unit where I had been a patient on bed rest for fifty days - the High Risk Obstetrics unit at Greater Baltimore Medical Center. I enjoy working with all the high risk moms. At first, it was therapeutic for me. Sharing my experience with my patients was cathartic. Then I began to realize that I had more to offer than good nursing care. I had practical advice and proof that a high risk pregnancy, even on bed rest, could be survived. Coworkers began telling me that I should write it down. So, here it is.

I wrote this guide to assist mothers-to-be to survive an abnormal pregnancy experience of bed rest, strained relationships, isolation, increased financial and emotional stress, and boredom. I've included some medical information but refer the reader to other sources for details and to the patient's doctor for personal instructions. I've shared my journal and my coping techniques in hopes that other high risk moms might more easily survive this bedrest before baby.

April 9, 1987
27 weeks

Dearest tiny one:

I love you. Your Daddy loves you. We can't wait to see you, to hold you in our arms. But for now, we hope you wait to arrive until a safer time. You are now just 27 weeks gestational age. You are not due to arrive until July 8. Since you've been threatening to debut for several weeks, I've been on bedrest. Back in February, the doctors (Zern and Facciolo) sutured my cervix and prescribed Terbutaline to delay labor. However, last Friday, (4/3) I became sick (a virus?) and the vomiting irritated the uterus which started contracting up to every five minutes. At that point Dad brought me to the Greater Baltimore Medical Center. Here they gave me IV Ritodrine which did not help. So they tried magnesium sulfate - a lot of it ... but it worked. Since Saturday morning I have been here on bedrest and taking Terbutaline again. The doctors want me to stay here until your arrival or at 34 weeks (7 weeks from now which is Memorial Day weekend), whichever occurs first.

I have such mixed feelings. I'm extremely anxious, as I said, to hold you, to see you, to know you're healthy. But I know that the best way to see you healthy is to wait as long as possible. The Lord knows when the time is best. We'll do our best to wait until that time.

I have so much to tell you. Where do I start? We know, from experience, that waiting is better because your brother, Christopher, was born at 31 weeks. He had a rough start, but he's hale and hearty now. I'm not sure what he thinks of my behavior. He's just 16 months old, so it's hard to say how much he understands. He's a very happy adaptable boy - I'm sure he'll be fascinated by you.

I know your oldest brother, Matthew, is already intrigued. He'll be 4 in July (Will you wait until then?). He listens to and feels my abdomen so he can hear you and feel you "kick". He prays daily that "God won't let the baby come too soon ... after summertime!" (a little too long, but he's got the idea).

1

Daddy is most cautious. He's the best Daddy in the world! He'll be ready for a vacation when you come. He has to work fulltime, keep the house running, take care of your brothers and worry about how you and I are doing. But he's not complaining at all. Like I said - he's the Best!

He does have a lot of help - we've been blessed with many loving and supportive friends and family. Grandmom visits me on her lunch hour, watches the guys on weekends and evenings so Dad can visit us. She also does our laundry, ironing, and some housecleaning, too! You've got a great Grandmom, too!

So many people are helping by watching Matthew and Christopher during the week that I have to keep track of them all on the calendar - Michael's cousin, his aunt, my Mom's cousin, Matthew's Sunday School teacher, a friend's mom, a babysitting co-op mom, women from church, and more! Friends from where I worked sent meals. We've had innumerable notes, prayers, balloons, and flowers from other friends, from church, from our Marriage Encounter Spiral. Your arrival is greatly anticipated by all. The Lord must have great plans for you. Let's not start too soon.

I enjoy feeling you inside of me. Every moment makes me smile. I feel very special to be blessed with you.

I love you,
Mom
****
April 10, 1987
27 2/7 weeks

Dear little one:

Today was a warm (70°) sunny spring day outside. Your Dad's feeling better and looks more rested. Matthew and Christopher were here to visit this evening. Matthew laid his ear to my abdomen to "hear the baby kick." He is anxious to have his Mom home soon.

We've had a lot more contractions today than we did yesterday. And I can feel you moving lower in my pelvis. I hope this doesn't mean you'll be forced out too soon. I have been concerned today. I am comforted though by the reassurance that the Lord will see us both safely through this journey. Be patient.

I love you,
Mom

****

April 11, 1987
27 3/7 weeks

I'm feeling very homesick tonight. Your Dad came to visit tonight by himself. He spent most of the time with his hand on my abdomen so he could feel you move. He thinks you're terrific.

Dad is feeling much better and looks well rested. He took a nap with Matthew and Christopher this afternoon. I miss them all so much and want to be at home with all of us together. But we must be patient. We love you and want you here safely.

Love,
Mom

****

April 13, 1987
27 5/7 weeks
11:30 PM

Dear little one:

We're getting closer!

Yesterday we were visited by friends from our old neighborhood, and Aunt Amy and Uncle Rick and, of course, Dad. We also got flowers from church. I have a new supply of books to read, needlework to do, and even ceramics (the Nativity set I started when Dad and I were first married).

You've been extremely active today. It feels great! Matthew was delighted to feel you "kicking" his hand tonight. So was Dad. Christopher was not paying attention, however.

We also saw Grandmom (at lunchtime). A priest from her parish visited today. And Pastor Klein brought Communion to me. My spirits were lifted by all these visits and with the knowledge that we are a few days closer to your safe arrival.

Are you a boy or a girl? I often wonder. It would be nice if you're a girl since we already have two boys ... then again, the boys are so much fun that a third would be nice, too. I am more concerned that you be healthy. Which name would you prefer? Michelle Denise or Patrick William?

Michelle - the feminine of your Dad's name
Denise - my middle name and a favorite of your Dad's
Patrick - masculine of my name, "noble"
William - a family name - your great-grandfather's name, Uncle John's middle name, my godfather's (Uncle Bill Miller) name.

I hope you'll like the one appropriate for your gender!

Sleep peacefully!

Love,
Mom

****

April 17, 1987
28 2/7 weeks
6:00 PM

Dearest baby:

You've moved! I mean you changed position. Your head is not in my pelvis, not pressing on my cervix. You are now lying transverse (horizontal). And you are growing. I've (we've) gained three pounds since last Tuesday. And we made it past 28 weeks!

I've only had two contractions so far today.

Last night, I was allowed up in a wheelchair to visit the Nursery and NICU with Matthew and Dad. (Christopher stayed with a friend from work last night - see why below). Matthew could only look through the windows at the babies because he wouldn't put a gown on. Peggy Eifert, Matthew's Sunday School teacher and a nurse here at the hospital, gave Matthew (and Christopher) some of her homemade Easter chocolates.

Today, Matthew had tubes put in his ears (myringotomies) at another hospital - he did real well - was anxious to get to McDonald's soon after.

Grandmom and her parish priest both visited again today. Pastor Don (Beutel) was here yesterday. Our best friends from our old neighborhood visited Wednesday night, while Dad took a break and went bowling.

I guess I'm learning to live at a "leisurely" pace. I've been fairly content to read and do some correspondence, some needlework. I feel much better about your safe arrival now that things have calmed down.

I received another injection of betamethasone to help mature your lungs (today).

Aunt Mary Ellen took Christy, your cousin, and Matthew to the movies (Disney's Aristocats) this afternoon. He's had a full day. He's enjoying this time of visiting with others while I'm here, but he's ready for me to come home ("in two minutes, O.K., Mom?").

I was very anxious about the boys on Wednesday without cause. They stayed with Jean Harberts and her boys, Kyle and Zachary. I knew Jean only as the Mom of Zachary, who was in St. Michael's nursery with Christopher. But I needn't have worried - Kyle and Matthew were instant friends. "He has trains and a little baby brother - just like me!" (Kyle is also 3 1/2 years old, Zach is one year old).

Dad is coming to visit by himself tonight. I miss him so much. I need his hugs! We'll be glad to be home all together as a family. (But we can wait - don't hurry!)

Take care in there!

I love you,
Mom

April 19, 1987
28 4/7 weeks

Happy Easter Little One!

Spring, Resurrection, New Life, Your Life - all beginning. God's Gifts, You, Matthew, Christopher - all so unique, so special, so miraculous!

Dad brought the guys in after church - both dressed in navy blue pants, white shirts, with blue bow ties, and Kelly green jackets. They are so handsome. So is your dad!

(Dad is feeling better ... getting over the cold.)

Matthew called excitedly this morning to tell me "the Easter Bunny left me a basket!" He told me about how he and Dad had dyed eggs yesterday. They had a good time.

Then they left here, they went to Grandmom's for dinner and the Easter Egg Hunt with everybody else (John and Barbara, Amy and Rick, Mary Ellen, Dan, and Christy).

Dad came back alone to visit later while Grandmom took care of the boys.

Dad says that when Matthew is frustrated, he occasionally says, "I'll never see Mom again." It's been such a long time for him that I've not been home. I'm sure he's confused, maybe angry that I "left him". I know that he knows something about your coming and that we have to wait "'til it's safe." I'm not sure how much to make of this or quite what, if anything, I should do. Maybe I'll talk with Dr. Zern tomorrow. She, being a mom and an M.D. might have some insight. You seem to be doing very well. You are active. Your heartbeat is 150-160 b.p.m. (a girl, according to old wives' tales).

Dad took a picture of me today. My "official pregnant picture." So you can see how we looked <u>before</u> delivery.

Praise the Lord for all His blessings!

Love,
Mom

****

April 23, 1987
29 1/7 weeks
10:00 PM

Dear Olympic hopeful:

You have been extremely active in the last two days! Yesterday, you kicked so hard I thought you would push out right through my abdomen. Today, I frequently felt you push on my cervix. I had quite a few contractions last night. They stopped just before I needed to go on the monitor. Slow down, little one, I know we got past 28 weeks but we can wait a little longer, can't we?

Dad brought the boys in tonight. Christopher is now standing alone more frequently, for longer periods. Matthew seems to be doing well. He's stopped saying he'll never see me again. I didn't get to talk to Dr. Zern, but I did speak with Dr. Machiran about Matthew. He said it's normal behavior - he'd be concerned if he were apathetic, withdrawn, or abusive. He also reminded me that when I do get home, I'll be adding insult to injury by bringing you home, too ... that you will require much of my time and attention. Therefore, Matthew will not get as much as he did before. He suggested we bring him a gift from you at that time - got any special gifts in mind?

I did reassure Matthew that I will be home after you arrive, that it may seem like a long time, but he can visit and call frequently.

I have kept busy by addressing Uncle John and Aunt Barbara's wedding invitations, by addressing shower invitations, by finishing a friend's needlework, by reading, and by being visited: Grandmom, Pastor Klein (who encouraged my writing about this experience), friends from our old neighborhood, Uncle John, Aunt Barbara, and of course, Dad, Christopher, and Matthew.

I'm very anxious about your activity, the contractions, and mostly the cervical pressure. I am not sure I an ready to deliver you. I'm scared and nervous - Will I be up to the experience - the pain,

the unknown? I want to be awake, I'd like for you to arrive naturally.
I know God will give us the strength we need.

Dad will be ready (camera and all), I think. He would like
you to wait a few more weeks. Take care!

I love you,
Mom
****
April 24, 2987
29 2/7 weeks
10:30 PM

Dear Impatient One:

Last night was another active one! More frequent
contractions and lots of cervical pressure resulted in my being placed
in Trendelenburg position (feet, hips elevated - to get pressure off my
cervix). It worked, but I had much difficulty getting to sleep.

I prayed for strength and peace. I thought about Pastor
Klein's encouragement to write about us and came up with a start.
I plan to start òn it tonight.

Dad visited with the guys. We shared some fruit and some
drawing. Dad took some more pictures of all of us.

I hope this is an uneventful night. I'm not sure I'm ready
yet. Oh yes, Grandmom was here at lunchtime, and Pastor Don also
visited and brought materials to make banners for Marriage
Encounter. I started on them this evening - just attached the
hangers.

I also prepared the bill payments and cards for the month.

You can see I'm keeping busy, please be patient.

Love,
Mom

April 27, 1987
29 5/7 weeks
11:00 PM

Dear Little One:

I miss the rest of the family. Dad came by himself Saturday night. We had a "date night" complete with popcorn and Coke. It was a nice evening.

Unfortunately, Matthew was sick on Sunday morning. He vomited all day. He seemed better by 6:00 PM ... but he was still lethargic. Monday, he was grumpy. When Dad got home from work today, he had a fever (102°). Dad took him to Dr. Jodorkovsky to check his ears. His ears were okay - "just a virus". So he's home drinking fluids and taking Tylenol. I hope he's okay in the morning and I hope Christopher and Dad don't get it.

I want to be home to take care of them all. Dad's great. He just keeps reminding me of my important job - keeping you inside to grow and develop as much as possible. Do your job - grow and develop!

We're doing okay - almost 30 weeks! See you soon (not too soon).

Love,
Mom
****
May 2, 1987
30 3/7 weeks

Dear Baby:

It's May? And we've made it past 30 weeks ... not without incident. We spent Thursday night (actually Friday morning from 12:30 to 5:30 AM) in the Delivery Room being monitored and given IV fluids to slow down the contractions (every seven minutes). It worked and we came back to room 2615 at 5:30-6:00 AM I was very tired - slept from breakfast until lunch on Friday.

Matthew is much better - if he stays well through the night Dad will bring the boys to visit tomorrow evening. I can't wait to see them! Dad couldn't bring them earlier this week 'cause Matthew had a relapse on Thursday (more vomiting and diarrhea). Christopher seems to be immune so far.

We have our first picture of you! A sonogram. You must be camera shy... at least you were not cooperative during the sono exam. When the technician tried to visualize your head, you had your hands in the way. Your arms were crossed over your chest and abdomen making it difficult to see your stomach. And when he tried to measure your leg bones (for growth), you kicked incessantly.

I saw your tiny heart beating. It's so hard to connect the image on the screen with a new person - you! But it's our first glimpse - like a sneak preview. We still don't know if you are Michelle or Patrick, but we do know that you weigh about 1700 grams (over 3 lbs.). And growing on schedule. (I've gained only 13 pounds - I think I've lost muscle by resting so much). I'm saving your sono picture for your scrapbook.

The sono took 45 minutes to complete. Then, in the afternoon, I heard about Matthew's relapse. I cried because I wanted to be with him, because I missed all the guys, because I was disappointed that I'd have to wait another few days to see them. I guess that the stress of the day could've exacerbated the contractions which took us to the DR (delivery room). I was afraid they would have to use Mag Sulfate again, but things calmed down. The Lord is watching over us.

Pastor Don was in on Friday afternoon. He helped to cheer me up. But Dad's surprise visit at lunchtime had really perked me up. (He was en route between the airport and Hunt Valley offices of Westinghouse for work). Your Dad is so special! He's not just surviving this, he's doing all of the little things that make the boys and me feel so important, so uniquely loved.

I love him. I love the boys. I love you. I yearn to hold you all closely.

God has given us this special time to learn new roles, to appreciate each member of our family. Let's thank Him.

Love,
Mom

May 6, 1987, Wednesday
31 weeks!

Who"d have thought we'd make it to 31 weeks!?! This is
great! I think ... I mean ... I'm so thankful to have made it so far, but
I'm tired of this life-style. I'm ready (for me) for this time to be
over ... to be able to do so many little loving acts. "There's no place
like home."

I've been having contractions more often, more frequently,
closer together, but no pressure or increased intensity. The
terbutaline doesn't seem to be as effective as it had been. I wonder
how much longer it will hold.

This morning I awoke at 4:00 AM with a contraction. I
had been dreaming that I had been having frequent contractions. I
wasn't sure if I had only dreamed them or if I had actually had them.
It was disquieting. I took my Terbutaline and went back to sleep
with no more contractions.

Later, Dr. Facciolo said, "Just don't dream yourself into
labor."

Dad visited with the guys last night. They are all so
handsome and loving. I miss them so.

Aunt Doris and Uncle Stanley also dropped in.

Grandmom continues to visit every lunchtime.

Pastor Klein brought Communion yesterday It is renewing
to have such contact with God and the church. This time doesn't
seem like a problem at all when compared to Jesus' sacrifice for us.
We are truly a blessed family to have each other with such minor
tribulations. (Please, Lord, help me to remember this when I feel so
ready to complain and also, Lord grant me patience and I need it
now!)

I also need a new "project". I've been doing crossword
puzzles. It passes the time but I'd like to feel more useful.

I've learned so many lessons which I need to remember when I go back to work:

✓ Patients do need to feel useful, active.

✓ I need to anticipate needs, comfort measures, to encourage patients to ask for the little things I wouldn't otherwise think of.

✓ To involve the patient more in deciding on time schedules, and routines, to adapt nursing assessments and actions to the patients' needs even more than I did before.

✓ To check each patient at least once an hour for assessment and to meet patients' social interaction needs.

I hope I don't forget.

****

May 9, 1987
31 3/7 weeks
1:30 PM

Dear One:

The last few days have been uneventful - a few contractions here and there but no pattern.

Matthew and Christopher are both well and have visited the last two nights. Today they are visiting with Dave and Debbie and Gregory Stewart. Everyone who has taken care of them has told me that they are both very good. They have been through a lot and seem to be doing very well.

Dad will be in to visit after he goes to Walt and Darlene Greif's wedding (at 2:00 PM). This morning he mowed the lawn and planted the garden. It is sunny today ... supposed to be 80 degrees.

I have finished painting all the nativity scene except the camels and I have run out of brown paint. I'll have to wait until someone can get more for me. The only other thing to do today is watch TV (nothing on) or read. I could get bored at this rate.

Except - it's fun to feel you move inside of me - pushing and turning. I'll miss all your movement inside when you're here to be held in our arms. I'm excited because I know the time is near but

I'm still a little scared of delivery. Lord, give us the strength, faith, and peace we'll need.

Love,
Mom

****

May 13, 1987
32 weeks!
11:00 PM

Dearest One:

I'm afraid it is I who am losing patience. Monday night I told your dad I was very ready for you to arrive. I told him I felt like refusing the terbutaline and taking up horseback riding to encourage labor. I guess I feel safer ... that you will be healthy now that we've passed the time when Christopher was born ... and since, in addition, we have had five injections of dexamethasone to increase the rate of lung maturity.

Dad is ready to end his role of superparent. Dad says: Since God knows our limits and won't give us more than we can handle - surely we must be close to your arrival.

Christopher is officially walking. He really took off on Mother's Day (May 10). He grins and waits for everyone to notice his accomplishment, too.

Matthew, who has become a real chatterbox, has great plans for us. "After the baby comes, we come and take you home in the car and we put the baby in the back ... we have a party and Gregory and Josh and Jenna and Christy will come and play!"

Both boys need to get their hair cut soon ... before Uncle John's wedding. (I hope you and I are both there).

Dad is enjoying his new job - he sees the opportunity for his own growth and advancement. I'm happy for him and proud of him. I hope I can relieve him of some domestic duties soon, so he can spend more energy on work and more time at home to relax with us.

Hope to see you soon!

Love,
Mom

****

May 16, 1987, Saturday
32 3/7 weeks
8:00 PM

Dear Little One (who is getting bigger every day!):

We're on our way to 33 weeks! Have had some contractions but not intense or regular. Last night, I had a dream that the membranes ruptured but then I woke up. I had difficulty getting to sleep last night - tossed and turned most of the night. Now I'm tired ... hope I can sleep better tonight.

Well, I just finished painting the last figure in the nativity set. Dad took all but this last piece home this afternoon. He also took the Boston fern and some other things. He's hoping we'll be home real soon. Dr. Facciolo said this morning that she plans to increase my activity slightly and slowly this week in anticipation of discharging me next week ... maybe.

I'm beginning to get depressed about being here so long and on bedrest. I guess I need a new project ... but I am not really interested in doing anything here ... but having a baby and taking you home. I'm also getting nervous 'cause I don't want to miss John's wedding.

The shower for Barbara went well today. Christopher slept through it. Matthew ate and talked with everyone. Dad came to visit by himself. I was glad to see him, I wanted him to take me home, too! I wish I knew the Lord's plan for us. I guess I have to keep hanging in here. Waiting is not always fun.

Love,
Mom

May 20, 1987
33 weeks!

Dear Young One!

33 weeks! It's hard to believe we made it this far. I'm ready for you to come anytime now.

Today I was allowed to get up, sit up, and walk a little. This, in anticipation of going home on Sunday. It felt good to walk even a little. My legs are wobbly and weak but working fairly well. My outlook is a little cheerier - just knowing that something will be happening by Sunday. Dad is glad to see some hope, too.

Today is Grandmom's birthday. Dad brought us some ice cream last night to share today at lunch. Grandmom is busy at work and at home with the wedding coming soon. She's bringing me some more to do - now I'm framing her needlework pieces. It helps pass the time.

The nursing staff gave me a huge balloon (approximately two feet in diameter) to "celebrate" seven weeks of time here (and to cheer us up). It happens to be pink ... but they say they hadn't thought about that - are you a girl or boy? I can't wait to see you!

Dad was here alone tonight - we had a chance to relax and talk. It felt so good to have him nearby. It's difficult to talk now when the boys come. Christopher is no longer content to stay in this room - he wants to walk - up and down the hall. So Michael walks with him while I visit with Matthew. We color, read, chat and polish (and "unpolish") his nails.

Hope to be home soon!

Love
Mom

May 23, 1987, Saturday
33 3/37 weeks
9:00 AM

We're Going Home!

No contractions, still haven't ruptured membranes ...

Dad will be here to pick us up about 11:00 AM I can't wait. We still have to stay on bedrest at home but at least we'll be home ... I can feel Dad lying next to me at night, I can play with the boys anytime, I can watch them grow - it happens so quickly. I can get outside, if only on the patio. This is great!

I guess you're going to wait a little while. I hope until after June 6 - Uncle John's wedding.

Love,
Mom

****

May 25, 1987, Monday
33 5/7 weeks

Well, we've been home for almost three days ... so far no rupture, a few contractions.

It is so nice to be home. It is great to be with Dad and the boys so much.

Christopher is walking everywhere - pushing his "corn popper". He gets frustrated easily - if he falls or if his way is obstructed.

Matthew and I have had several long talks about you. That it has been "a lot of trouble" to get you here, that we'd like to see you soon, that he wants to do more things than he can now because of "the baby," he tickles you, feels you move, says you giggle when tickled. He's very moody, sensitive since I've been home. It must be a most confusing time for him. We need to pray for him.

I think we're all worn out emotionally and ready for you.

Hope to see you soon,

Love,
Mom
****

July 26, 1987
5 2/7 weeks old!

Dear <u>Patrick</u>!

It's hard to believe you're over five weeks old already. Things have been extremely busy since June 19th. Let me fill you in.

I came home on bedrest at 33 weeks. I stopped taking the terbutaline at 36 weeks. I had continued to have frequent mild contractions after discharge. These increased in frequency a little after stopping the medicine. I also continued to gain weight. I began to wonder if I'd ever go into true labor.

On June 18, I took Matthew and Christopher up to see Daddy working on the trees at his cousin's new house (they had cut down six old trees and were cutting and splitting.) We took your cousins to get snowballs. On the ride back I noticed I was more uncomfortable but this had become the norm. That night, Dad got home at about 10:00 PM and we got to bed at about 11:00 PM

At 12:30 AM on June 19 I awoke with a start and a strong contraction. Then I had cramps and felt some fluid leaking. I went to the bathroom - fluid continued leaking just a little ... I had a BM and then stopped cramping and leaking. I thought, at first, that maybe it was another false alarm. I went back to bed. After just a few minutes I knew you were on your way - I began to have very strong contractions every five minutes.

I called Dr. Facciolo and Grandmom. Grandmom came over to sit with Matthew and Christopher and Dad drove us to the hospital. We arrived at 1:10 AM and on admission exam learned that I was 3 c.m. dilated. By 2:30 AM I was 6 c.m. dilated and I wanted to push.

At 3:09 AM, after just three pushes (and a lot of encouragement and support from Dad, Dr. Facciolo, and the nurse), you were born!

The cord was around your neck, so Dr. Facciolo had to loosen and move it, but there were no complications!

You are gorgeous - you had lots of blond hair, were red and wrinkled, and cried lustily! I loved you instantly (though I've been loving you sight unseen for months.) Dad held you and I held you and nursed you then Dr. Facciolo cut the cord, delivered the placenta, stopped the bleeding and sutured a few cervical tears and the episiotomy. Then we held you again and hesitantly handed you to the nurse. You were taken to the nursery for evaluation and bathing . I was taken to Room 2537 and rested for a few hours.

I called some people to tell them about you and Dad went home to get some rest and to care for the other boys.

We came home on June 21 (after checking your bilirubin level of 11.5)

Matthew and Christopher want to hold, hug, and kiss you all the time. They love you.

For the past month I have been learning to juggle my time and energies amongst the three of you and Daddy.

You've been such a good baby. The second week you were sleeping 6-7 hours at night (almost every night).

Neither of the boys seems truly jealous of you. Though Christopher wants to sit on my lap while I nurse you.

They do compete against each other for your attention (and mine).

Christopher is running everywhere. He has also learned to bite Matthew. (He's learning that is not permissible, also).

Matthew had his fourth birthday (got his Hot Wheels train - what else?) and is learning to be more independent every day. He's looking forward to preschool. He starts at the Perry Hall Children's Center on September 9th.

We went to the fireworks at Fullerton for the Fourth of July - actually we sat on the parking lot of ValuFood but we saw and heard them without fighting crowds and noise.

We saw Dr. Machiran on July 11th, Saturday morning. Matthew had his preschool exam and DTP and polio. You had a four week exam and PKU. You were 7 lbs. 1 oz. and 21 inches long. You are growing so quickly.

I will be returning to work on Wednesday, July 29 if my six week exam is okay as I expect it will be. I'll be working when Dad is home - no sitters - one weekend shift and one evening (5:00 to 11:30 PM) each week at the same hospital where I worked before bedrest.

Praise God - all is settling into routine at the Isennock's!

Praise the Lord for you - you are truly a miraculous gift to us. I know He will give us the wisdom and guidance we'll need to help you grow as a Christian.

I now hold you and know you must weigh over 8 lbs. I marvel at the perfectness of your body. From your tiny toes to your blond locks. I'm amazed at your abilities and alertness. We all love you.

I'm going to start to put your baby book together (if I have the time).

I love you Patrick William!

Love,
Mom

P.S. We did attend Uncle John's wedding on June 6 when you were 36 weeks gestational age. It was beautiful!

I. "LET'S NOT START TOO SOON."

An incompetent cervix and preterm labor (PTL) were the causes of my required bedrest, but there are many reasons why your obstetrician may have ordered you to bed. And you are not alone!

High risk expectant mothers are advised to rest in various positions for varying reasons. Among the causes of pregnancy bedrest are:

* placenta previa
* preterm labor
* premature rupture of membranes (PROM)
* multiple fetuses (twins, triplets,...)
* pregnancy-induced hypertension (PIH - previously known as preeclampsia or toxemia)
* gestational diabetes

Bedrest is beneficial in all of these cases because it increases the blood supply to the baby and decreases physical stresses on the mother. Additionally, bedrest is known to lower blood pressure and enhance kidney function.[1] The goal is to maintain the best possible environment in which your baby can grow and develop. Your job, then, is to be an incubator!

My job as incubator was made easier to accept since we had seen, firsthand, the results of not incubating long enough. Our second son, Christopher, was born without warning at 31 weeks. Fortunately, he suffered no major life-threatening consequences. Still, he remained in the Neonatal Intensive Care Unit (NICU) for over a month and, due to a digestive disorder, he required special feedings and an apnea monitor for almost a year. It was a traumatic, sleepless, and financially devastating experience we did not wish to repeat. The advanced technology found in NICU's has significantly decreased the numbers of deaths and the frequency of brain damage in prematurely delivered babies. But the best of hi-tech equipment cannot usually match the benefits of good prenatal care.[2] And the cost of even hospitalized bedrest during pregnancy is only a fraction of the cost of NICU care of a preterm infant.[3]

Perhaps your job as an incubator might be made easier with more information about the cause of your need for pregnancy bedrest. For each of the common causes I will explain what it is,

21

how it is diagnosed, how it is managed by health personnel, what you can do about it, and the possible outcomes. This book is not intended to be a medical guide, so I will also tell you where you can find more information about each condition. Please be sure to ask your doctor for specific advice for your situation.

Placenta Previa

Placenta previa occurs when the placenta is implanted near or over the internal os, the opening of the cervix. This appears to happen in 0.4 - 0.6% (or 1/260 -1/167) of all pregnancies.[4] There are varying degrees of previa and the status of previa may change at any time during a pregnancy. Total placenta previa describes a placenta which completely covers the cervical os. A partially covered os is called partial placenta previa. If the edge of the sac is just near the edge of the opening it is called marginal placenta previa. A low-lying placenta is in the lower segment of the uterus but does not touch the opening. As the baby grows and as the cervix dilates, a low-lying placenta may become a marginal, partial, or even total placenta previa.

The exact cause of placenta previa is not known. A large placenta, such as with twins or triplets, may approach or cover the os as it fills the uterus. Associated factors are those which may cause scar tissue in the uterine lining or that interfere with the blood supply to the uterine lining. These factors include: abortion, caesarean delivery, prior placenta previa, uterine infection, multiple pregnancies, closely spaced pregnancies, uterine tumors, and maternal age over 35.[5]

The first, most common symptom of previa is sudden painless bleeding which usually first occurs after the third month of pregnancy. The bleeding usually stops by itself but may start again at any time for no apparent reason. The doctor will most likely order an ultrasound exam (sonogram) to locate the position of the placenta. He will probably not do a cervical exam since this may aggravate the bleeding.

Medical management of placenta previa depends upon the maturity and welfare of the baby and upon the extent of bleeding. If the baby is premature and the bleeding is not severe, delivery may be delayed. The mother may be placed on bedrest to maintain the blood supply to the baby at the best level possible while decreasing the chances of hemorrhage. She may be hospitalized to allow for close observation of the bleeding and frequent monitoring of the baby. An intravenous (IV) line may be kept open in the event that she might need extra fluids or blood. Blood may be drawn each day to monitor the mother's blood count. The baby will be evaluated by the use of fetal activity charts, electronic fetal monitoring, and by nonstress tests. These are discussed in detail in the next chapter. Due to the potential for hemorrhage, the baby is usually delivered by caesarean section.

Preterm Rupture of Membranes (PROM)

Preterm rupture of membranes occurs when the amniotic sac in which the baby is growing, breaks open and amniotic fluid may leak out. Though this usually occurs spontaneously during labor, the cause of premature rupture is not clear. It may or may not be associated with preterm labor. PROM is verified by a vaginal exam for the presence of amniotic fluid. This fluid can be distinguished from normal vaginal discharge by the use of Nitrazine paper which turns dark blue in the presence of amniotic fluid. Thus, if the Nitrazine test is positive, PROM is confirmed.

Ultrasound exams (sonograms) may be done to determine the baby's gestational age, to locate the position of the baby, and to assess the volume of amniotic fluid. If the baby is mature and labor has begun, it is allowed to progress and the baby is delivered. If the baby is premature but not in distress and the mother is not in labor, she may be kept in the Labor and Delivery area or transferred to a High Risk Obstetrical Unit for close monitoring. She will be observed for signs of labor and/or infection. The baby will be monitored for level of maturity and signs of distress.

If the mother is in labor and the baby is premature, but not in distress, the labor may be delayed by bedrest, fluids, and medications. These are discussed under Preterm Labor. If the mother is in labor and the baby is premature and in distress, the baby is delivered and cared for in a Neonatal Intensive Care Unit.

Preterm Labor

Most people consider preterm labor to be any labor which begins at any time prior to the baby's due date. A strict medical definition would define preterm labor as regular uterine contractions after 20 weeks and before 37 weeks which are 5-8 minutes apart or less and accompanied by cervical dilatation and/or effacement. Approximately 8% of all pregnancies end in preterm labor. The cause cannot be identified in over 50% of these cases but the list of associated risk factors is a long one which includes:

> prior preterm labor
> low socioeconomic status
> low maternal weight gain
> smoking
> mother less than 18 or greater than 40 years old
> heavy work
> exposure to diethylstilbestrol (DES) during
>   pregnancy of the patient's mother
> infections of the urinary tract, vagina, or uterus
> uncontrolled diabetes
> twins, triplets, etc.
> incompetent cervix
> preterm rupture of membranes
> placenta previa
> fetal distress
> fetal malformations
> fetal growth retardation (baby not growing
>   appropriately)
> fetal death

The first decision to be made in the medical management of PTL is whether delaying labor and delivery of the baby would be beneficial or harmful. Prolonging the pregnancy may be harmful in cases of fetal death, fetal malformations, fetal distress, fetal growth retardation, or infection. Delaying labor may be helpful if the baby is premature but not in distress.

Once the decision is made to attempt to prolong the pregnancy, the mother is placed on bedrest, usually in a side-lying or Sims position, to enhance the blood supply to the baby. A Trendelenburg position may be prescribed if there is pressure from the baby on the cervix which is causing dilatation, effacement, or contractions. This position requires the pelvis to be elevated above the level of the shoulders and head. This position uses gravity to relieve cervical pressure. Hospital beds can easily be placed in this position. At home, Trendelenburg may be achieved by placing blocks under the foot supports of the bed or by the use of a dense foam rubber wedge cut to the doctor's specifications.

Dehydration is avoided by encouraging fluids. Bedrest may be maintained at home with frequent checkups and/or at-home electronic monitoring, or in the hospital. The mother is advised to refrain from douching, having intercourse, and preparing her nipples for breast-feeding by nipple-rolling. These activities may stimulate labor. It may be necessary to start an intravenous (IV) line to maintain an adequate fluid level. The mother is observed closely for signs of progressive labor and/or any complications. The baby is monitored for level of maturity and signs of distress.

Bedrest and fluids alone may not delay delivery, in which case any one or combination of medications may be used. These medications are classified as tocolytics, or labor suppressants. The earlier in labor that these medications are started the more successful they will probably be.[6] These medicines should not be used in cases of fetal growth retardation or uterine infection. They should be used cautiously, if at all, in the presence of placenta previa, rupture of membranes, diabetes, renal disease, or hypertension.

Ritodrine is the only drug approved by the Federal Drug Administration for use as a tocolytic. It slows the contractions of the uterus, and, therefore, delays labor. It is more expensive than some other tocolytics and does have some side effects. It increases the heart rates of both mother and baby, decreases the mother's blood pressure, and may cause apprehension, palpitations, chest tightness, headache, trembling, fever, nausea, vomiting, hallucinations, and electrolyte imbalances. Most people experience the less severe side effects to varying degrees. The more serious side effects are more rare.

Other medications, though not officially approved by the FDA for use as tocolytics, have been used on a regular basis. These drugs are approved by the FDA for other uses but have been found to be effective as tocolytics. Terbutaline, for example, is also known as Brethine and is used for asthma and respiratory diseases. It is useful, however, in decreasing contractions. It is less expensive than Ritodrine and causes fewer and less severe side effects. Trembling, shaking, headache, and palpitations are the most common complaints of patients. Increased heart rate also occurs. At first, the harder you try to control the trembling, the worse it becomes. After about a week of therapy, the trembling, shaking, and palpitations seem to decrease in severity. Terbutaline until just recently was given only by injection in an emergency or in pill form every four hours. A new innovation called the terbutaline pump, allows a steady continuous administration of the medication without interruption of the mother's sleeping hours. A very small pump is filled with terbutaline and programmed to deliver appropriate doses at scheduled times through a tiny tube into the skin. This method usually decreases "breakthrough" contractions which might otherwise occur just before a terbutaline pill is due since the mother's blood level of the medication is low at that time. The mother can be taught to maintain the pump either in the hospital or at home. Insurance coverage of the pump varies widely and may dictate when and in which situations it is utilized.

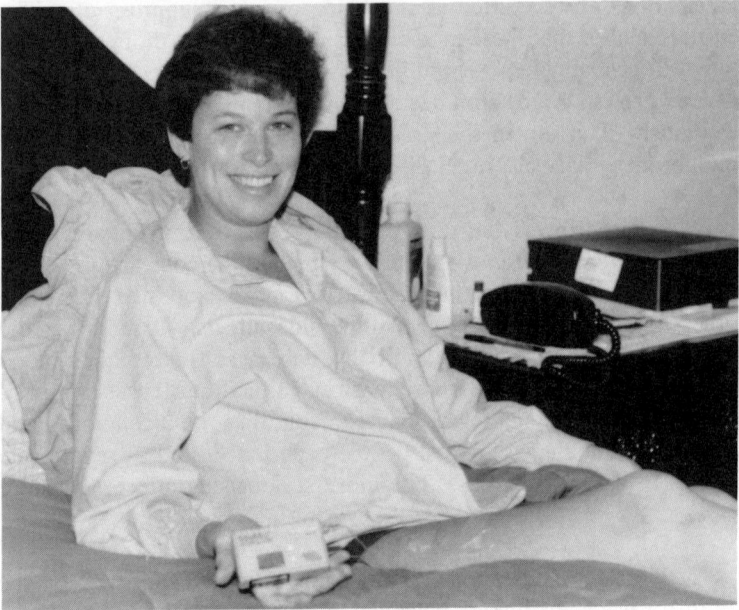

A Terbutaline Pump in use.

Magnesium sulfate was previously used in pregnancy only for patients with high blood pressure. Because it interferes with muscle contractions it has been used effectively as a tocolytic. Serious side effects are uncommon. It should not be used in patients with myasthenia gravis, poor kidney function, or recent heart attack. It does decrease blood pressure, muscle tone, and breathing rate. It does not affect the baby's heart rate. Common complaints include nausea, vomiting, headache, nasal congestion, and hot flushes. With larger doses, mag sulfate can cause more severe symptoms such as chest pain, shortness of breath, or feelings of paralysis. Most mothers who have experienced mag sulfate say they would rather deliver than to repeat the experience since it can be a quite frightening one. In reality, many mothers willingly tolerate a second round of the medication when premature labor threatens the life of their baby.

Other medications used as tocolytics include aspirin, indomethacin, nifedipine, and naproxen. These are not used as often, have more side effects, and do not seem as reliable for most patients.

Prolonging pregnancy, by whatever means, is done strictly to allow the baby to grow and develop to a point at which he or she could survive outside the womb. This ability to survive is most dependent upon the maturity of the baby's lungs. Maturation of the lungs requires the presence of a substance called surfactant which helps to keep the lungs from collapsing. Surfactant begins to appear at approximately 26 weeks and increases greatly at 32 weeks. The lack of surfactant is the major cause of Respiratory Distress Syndrome (RDS) or hyaline membrane disease (HMD) which is the major cause of premature infant death. Surfactant can now be administered to premature infants. This has decreased the incidence of HMD.

Allowing time for the formation of surfactant is a primary goal of delaying delivery. The formation of surfactant is actually accelerated by any factor which places stress on the baby These factors include: placenta previa, chronic kidney or cardiac disease, sickle cell disease, hyperthyroidism, heroin addiction, uterine infection, preterm labor, or rupture of membranes. Also, it has been found that the use of a medication called betamethasone within one week prior to delivery can decrease the chances of RDS significantly.[7,8] Betamethasone is a steroid drug and must be used with caution, especially in mothers who also have diabetes, pregnancy-induced hypertension, or who are also taking tocolytic medications. It may increase the risk of infection or slow healing of wounds. It is usually given once a week by injection. There appear to be no ill effects on the baby. At least one study has shown there were no differences in mental, verbal or visual abilities at four years of age in children who were exposed to betamethasone during pregnancy.[9]

Multifetal pregnancy

A multifetal pregnancy is the result of the fertilization of two or more eggs at the same time or of the fertilization of one egg which then divides into two similar eggs. The incidence of identical (from one egg) twins is approximately one set per 250 births. Dizygotic or fraternal (two or more eggs at the same time) twins occur more frequently, especially with the use of fertility drugs and in vitro fertilization (IVF). The exact incidence varies by race, heredity, age, and number of pregnancies.[10] Diagnosis can be made on the basis of the presence of two or more distinct heart sounds, by abnormally elevated growth hormone levels in the mother's blood, or by the presence of two sacs on ultrasound examination.

The medical management of multifetal pregnancy does not necessarily differ from that of a unifetal pregnancy in the first two trimesters. It is in the third trimester that controversy over management begins. Many studies have debated the benefits of bedrest in otherwise normal multifetal pregnancies.[11] Generally, however, it is agreed that bedrest begun at 28 weeks results in prolonged pregnancies, higher birth weights, fewer infant deaths, and fewer incidents of pregnancy-induced hypertension (PIH).[12] This bedrest usually occurs in the hospital to allow for close observation of both mother and babies.

Other complications of pregnancy, such as placenta previa, PIH, fetal growth retardation, preterm labor, and preterm rupture of membranes, occur more frequently in multifetal pregnancies and are treated as they occur.

Pregnancy-induced hypertension (PIH)

Pregnancy-induced hypertension is the latest medical terminology for what is commonly referred to as toxemia of pregnancy or preeclampsia. PIH is now diagnosed on the basis of a blood pressure greater than 140/90 (or a blood pressure which is significantly higher than the mother's usual pressure) and the presence of protein in her urine. Preeclampsia is now determined by increased blood pressure, protein in urine, and generalized swelling which occurs after 20 weeks. Eclampsia occurs when all of the above are present and the patient experiences convulsions. Early indications of PIH (high blood pressure and protein in urine) are usually not detected by the mother. Later signs, such as sudden weight gain due to fluid retention, headaches, problems with vision, and pain in the upper abdomen are usually not seen until the condition is serious.

PIH may be caused by an immune response, a sort of rejection of the placenta and fetus by the mother's body.[13] The predisposition for developing PIH is inherited. Approximately 5% of all pregnancies are complicated by PIH, though the incidence is higher in Black and Hispanic populations. Teens and mothers over 35 years of age also have a higher rate of PIH.[14] Left uncontrolled, PIH may result in eclampsia, kidney failure, placental abruption (separation of the placenta from the uterus), or stroke. Early detection and treatment, however, can minimize even the early signs of PIH.

Mothers who are diagnosed as having developed PIH will be asked to report any new symptoms such as headache, changes in vision, abdominal pain, weight gain, swelling, nausea, and/or vomiting. The doctor will want to check her urine for protein on a regular basis. He will also draw her blood to monitor her blood count and liver and kidney functions. She will be advised to stop smoking because smoking causes the blood vessels to tighten, which results in higher blood pressure.

In some cases, the mother is hospitalized for evaluation and possible treatment. If so, the nursing staff will closely monitor her and her baby. A complete assessment will be done at least once a shift (usually every eight hours). The nurse will check her temperature, blood pressure, and urine. She will ask if the patient has experienced any headaches, upper abdominal pain, or changes in her vision. The mother's reflexes will be checked, as they are a good indication of the severity of PIH. A record of the amounts of fluid the mother has drunk and the volume of urine excreted will be kept to detect any fluid retention early. For this same reason, the mother will be weighed daily.

The baby will be observed by use of electronic monitoring and ultrasound exams (sonograms). The baby's heart rate may be checked as often as every four hours. The mother will be asked to keep a record of the baby's activity level and to report any changes in activity.

The need to alter the diet of a mother with PIH is somewhat controversial. Some say protein and fluids should be increased while salt should be strictly limited.[15]   As a rule, PIH patients are instructed to drink 8-10 glasses of fluid each day and to eat a well-balanced diet. Some hypertensive mothers may be required to increase the amount of proteins to replace that which is lost in the urine. Others may be requested to limit salt intake to avoid fluid retention. Diuretics, or fluid pills, have not been found to be useful and may be harmful to the baby by decreasing the blood flow to the placenta.[16]

The most frequently used medication in the management of PIH is magnesium sulfate. This drug is used to avoid the possibility of convulsions, especially during labor and for the first twenty-four hours after delivery. The side effects include hot flashes, loss of muscle tone, nausea, vomiting, and nasal congestion. It does not affect the baby's heart rate. (See the discussion of magnesium sulfate under Preterm Labor.) Magnesium sulfate (also called mag sulfate) may be used in combination with high blood pressure medications, such as hydralazine, to control PIH and prevent complications. Some doctors may order a baby aspirin every day since some studies have shown that small doses of aspirin can decrease the incidence of preeclampsia.[17] Betamethasone may be used to aid the baby's lung development. (See discussion under Preterm Labor.)

Bedrest is essential for all mothers with PIH. Resting in bed on the left side takes the pressure of the baby off a major blood vessel, the inferior vena cava. As a result, swelling is decreased, blood pressure is lowered, kidney function is improved, and the blood supply to the baby is increased. Research has shown that bedrest can lower the possibility of infant death by 50%.[18] Most doctors will advise mothers with PIH to lie on their left side at all times except when using the bathroom.

PIH is temporary and is cured by delivery of the baby. If the condition is mild, most doctors will attempt to prolong the pregnancy to allow the baby's lungs to mature. But if symptoms become severe, the risks for both mother and baby increase. The chances for the baby's survival are then greater in a neonatal intensive care unit than in the mother's uterus. After delivery, the mother improves quickly and can be discharged without medication if her blood pressure is stable.

Gestational diabetes

Diabetes, caused by a pancreas which is not able to produce enough insulin, results in the improper use of fats and proteins for energy. Women who are pregnant and have diabetes can be divided into two groups: diabetics who became pregnant and pregnant women who became diabetic. Diabetics who become pregnant may need to adjust their diet and insulin needs frequently to adapt to the many physical and emotional changes of pregnancy. Occasionally, this adjustment process requires hospitalization for close observation of glucose levels.

Pregnant women who become diabetic are known as gestational diabetics. Reported rates of gestational diabetes vary widely from 0.15% to 12.3% of all pregnancies.[19] The differences may result from the criteria used for diagnosis. Although glucose tolerance testing is done routinely for prenatal care, the techniques used and the methods of evaluation vary. However the test is done, a consistently high glucose level in an otherwise normal pregnant woman is indicative of gestational diabetes. Pregnancy causes an increase in metabolic rate, an increase in physical stress, and some anti-insulin effects which can result in gestational diabetes for those at risk. Risk factors include : age greater than 30, a family history of diabetes, previous birth of a large infant, obesity, and hypertension. Uncontrolled gestational diabetes can result in many complications, some of which are: increased chance of preeclampsia, severe infections, large babies and difficult deliveries, increased chance of hemorrhage after delivery, infant death, congenital defects, and injury to baby during delivery.

Careful control of gestational diabetes can minimize the possibility of developing any complications. When the disorder is managed well the survival rate for infants of mothers with gestational diabetes is as good as that for any infants.[20] This management begins with monitoring the mother's blood glucose 2 or 3 times a day. Initially, this may require a brief hospital stay. While in the hospital, the patient is taught to test her own blood and urine for glucose and to adjust her activity, diet, and insulin dose accordingly. The goal of these modifications is to maintain the blood glucose at normal levels (80-120 mg./100 my.). The patient is also advised to report any signs of infection, or nausea and/or vomiting at any time during her pregnancy. She is requested to maintain a record of the baby's activity and to report any changes. The baby is also monitored by ultrasound exam and stress tests. No diabetic pills (oral hypoglycemics) are prescribed since these may be harmful to the baby.

Unless complications arise, the baby is usually delivered close to or on the due date. Fifty to eighty percent of diabetic mothers deliver by caesarean section, but if the conditions are favorable (baby is not too large, cervix is soft, effaced and dilated, and the baby's position is appropriate) vaginal delivery is possible. It is important to note that even though the baby may be large and healthy in appearance, he is still a newborn, possibly premature, who requires the special attention of experienced correlatives. This may mean the infant will be admitted to the neonatal intensive care unit. The mother may also need close observation after delivery, since, unlike PIH, delivery does not always cure the disorder. While most mothers' glucose levels will return to normal soon after delivery, it appears that the majority of gestational diabetics will eventually become overt, or regular, diabetics.[21]

What you can do:

☞ Relax! I know this sounds ridiculous if you've been in bed for even a few days. But before you can help yourself or your baby, you have to stop your mind from racing, get as much information as possible, and be able to think straight. So, close your eyes, take a deep breath through your nose, and slowly blow out through your mouth. Now, remember any method you have used in the past to relax. Use it! Use all of them if you must. If you can't think of anything, try reading about relaxation techniques or listening to relaxation tapes. Most local libraries have them or can get them for you. Have a friend pick them up for you.

☞ Ask! Ask about everything that pops into your head. Keep a pad of paper and a pencil handy to write down all questions. Then refer to these whenever you talk to your doctor. Be sure you understand the answer completely. Repeat the answers in your own words and/or demonstrate and ask if you are correct.

Ask the nurse, assistant, volunteer, housekeeper, or anyone involved, if daily activities must occur as they do or if there is any flexibility. For example, if you are prescribed terbutaline, it may be necessary that you take it every six hours. But the times can be altered slowly to adapt to your regular schedule. You can take it at ten p.m. and four a.m. if you want to go to sleep early. Or you can take it at midnight and six a.m. if you like to stay up to watch the late news.

Read more about your situation. Ask your librarian to find any information about high risk pregnancy, medications, or treatments. If you are in the hospital, the hospital librarian may be able to help you. One word of caution: Don't read more than you want to know. It may only cause you to worry unnecessarily. Your doctor should be able to answer specific questions for you. Or perhaps he will recommend a pamphlet or book to help. Always check with your obstetrician before changing any activity or therapy.

☞ Follow directions! I can't tell you how many patients I've seen who have been admitted to the High Risk OB Unit for bedrest who refuse to follow directions. If you are told to lie on your left side, that does not mean you do so for fifteen minutes or until your friend visits. It means you lie on your left side as much as is humanly possible until the doctor or nurse tells you otherwise. Your friends can move around your bed and sit on the other side, and you aren't fooling anyone by waiting until the nurse leaves the room to change position. There is a reason for the directions. If you don't understand, ask again. I'd like a penny for every time I've heard a nurse or doctor say, "If she doesn't want to listen, why is she here?"

☞ Get help! Accept all offers and search for more. You need other people to link you with the rest of the world and to help with some basic needs. Shortly after I was admitted to the hospital I encountered a major crisis. No one was available for a few days to care for my two sons. I fretted and fretted until I mentioned this to my pastor who said, "I've been waiting for you to ask! I told you a lot of people have been offering to help in any way." One mother of two young boys said the only thing she could offer was baby-sitting. It was the only thing I needed at the moment! Still, I was very hesitant to accept help from someone I didn't know that well. I'm glad I did. All four boys enjoyed their times together.

Most people would be glad to help if only they knew how. Tell them. Ask them to pick up and deliver, to baby-sit, to clean, to iron, to move things, to rub your back, to share lunch, or just to listen when you call. Need more ideas? Check chapters two and nine. I'm sure you'll think of more as the days pass.

☞ Contact "Sidelines", a national network of support groups for women experiencing complicated pregnancies. See Resources.

☞ Write it down! There is space here for you to keep track of your diagnosis, medications, and instructions. Writing it down will help you remember why you are on bedrest, what you can and cannot do, when to take your medicine, and how to follow directions.

Keeping a record of any symptoms is also beneficial. Specific written information will help you to be more objective. With concrete data your doctor can make better decisions regarding your care. Ask your doctor which symptoms you should call about immediately and which you should record for your next regular visit. Use the chart of symptoms at the end of this chapter or make your own to suit your needs.

You may also wish to keep a journal of activities, tests, feelings. This may be kept as a memento or used as a therapy to help you survive the boredom.

☞ Remember! You <u>are</u> doing something. You are giving your baby the best possible environment in which to grow and develop.

My reason for being on bedrest is:_____

_____

Date I started bedrest:_____

It all started when:_____

_____

_____

_____

My instructions for bedrest:_____

      Position: __Trendelenberg __Sims (which side?) _

                      __other _____

      Bathroom: __go to bathroom _bedpan only

                      __bathtub __shower __sponge bath

      Time off: __may walk (where, when, how long?) ___

                      _____

                      __may sit in chair (how long?) _____

Medications I am taking:

Name	Reason	Dose	Times

Diet I should follow:_____

_____

_____

_____

_____

Other instructions:_____

_____

_____

_____

Questions:_____

_____

_____

_____

Chart of Symptoms

I should call my doctor IMMEDIATELY if I have any of the following symptoms:

___vaginal bleeding

___vaginal discharge, leaking of fluid

___contractions:

- more than every ___ minutes

- more than ___ per hour

- very strong contractions

___abdominal pain

___headache

___blurred or changed vision

___blood sugar

- less than ___

- greater than ___

___fainting spells

___(other) _____

Date	Time	Activity	Symptoms
		(diet, medication physical activity baby's movements)	(contractions, pain, vaginal discharge, bleeding, change in vision, headache, blood sugar, etc.)

_____

_____

_____

_____

_____

_____

_____

_____

_____

_____

II. "GOOD-BYE, NORMAL PREGNANCY!"

Okay! So now you're resigned to the fact that you are on bedrest for most, if not the rest of this pregnancy. Is there any way to maintain some semblance of normalcy? Can you even have a semi-normal pregnancy? Well ... to some degree ... yes! But, you might have to work on it.

Let's start with you. You are pregnant and, therefore, have certain pregnancy rights. First, you maintain the right to announce your pregnancy. Though you won't be out wandering around your usual haunts, you can call or write to anyone and everyone. This is also a good chance to explain your absence and to invite phone calls, letters, and visits. This is also your opportunity to begin to accept help. Write down the name, address, and phone number of anyone who even vaguely extends an offer.

Second, you have the right to look pregnant. Okay, so your audience may be limited. That's no excuse for not looking and feeling your best. Ask your doctor whether you may take a shower or bath - when, how long, and how often. Enjoy the bath or shower if you are allowed. Make do with a basin of water if you must. Try to maintain your normal hygiene schedule, if possible. You will feel better.

Have someone assemble your hygiene and beauty care products in a basket to keep at your bedside. Don't forget: wet wipes, tissues, cotton swabs, powder, deodorant, lotion, perfume, cosmetics, comb, brush, hair curlers, and nail polish and remover. This is the time to call your Avon or Mary Kay representative. Have her visit and deliver catalogs. You can order for yourself and for gifts - birthdays, Christmas, etc.

Finally, you have the right to all the normal emotions and questions of any other pregnant woman. Ask a friend to buy or borrow a book about normal pregnancy and delivery. Or order from a local bookstore and have them deliver or mail it. Ask your doctor and/or nurse for pamphlets and books.

Obviously, preserving semi-normalcy requires that you have certain things within reach. Have someone help you set up your immediate surroundings with all your supplies at hand. Some things you might want nearby are:

* telephone, telephone book with yellow pages, personal phone number listing.
* bell or whistle to summon help - you might consider investing in an infant intercom (the two-way type)... you can use it for the baby later
* calendar, date book
* television and VCR with remote controls, if available. Some video stores will deliver tapes, popcorn, and even pizza! Caution: Plan your viewing or you could become a TV zombie.
* radio, CB monitor, tape player
* reading material: books, magazines, professional journals, newsletters, church bulletins. Make arrangements for someone to bring in your newspaper and mail during the day.
* water pitcher and cup, straws, Thermos of your favorite beverage
* cooler and hot plate if you're home alone all day or want the independence. A cup-at-a-time coffee maker also heats water for tea or hot chocolate
* writing surface, lap desk, tray
* stationery, stamps, pens, pencils, scrap paper, notebook
* journal
* crossword puzzles, word finds, dictionary
* menus from food establishments which deliver
* kids box (for your other children, small visitors, and you!) with crayons, books, water paints, small toys, travel-type games, board games

Once you've organized your surroundings, you can organize your time. Keeping a date book or calendar handy can help you plan your days. I know this may sound ridiculous to someone who has no place to go but that doesn't mean you have no one to see or nothing to do.

Plan to "get up" in the morning by freshening up as allowed. Wear those maternity clothes you bought! In the hospital? Who says you must wear their "gowns"? Even if your membranes have ruptured you can wear maternity tops at least. If you have not shopped in the maternity departments, now's your chance. Get catalogs, and mail-order. Accept friends' hand-me-downs. Ask a friend to check out consignment shops.

Eat at somewhat regular times. Plan lunch, dinner, or snacks with friends. Set "dates" with your husband - order dinner to be delivered, get a videotape. If you don't have a VCR, watch a TV movie or rent a portable VCR from a video store. Read through the week's TV listing and schedule your viewing times. Also try to schedule your bedtime. Take into account any required snacks or medication times. If you are in the hospital you should be able to work with your primary nurse to avoid being disturbed at night or on "dates".

Maintaining a routine will help you keep track of time and decrease the chances of depression. It helps to count down the days and gives you something to look forward to each day. Keep a calendar nearby. Chart out the rest of your pregnancy by weeks. Include tests, events, doctor's appointments, special occasions. Celebrate the completion of each week in a special way - a date night with Dad, a takeout meal, a visit with a close friend.

You will have good days and bad days in the next few weeks - some very good and some very bad. Hopefully the good days will outweigh the bad ones. Gina Robinson, a mother on bedrest for 10 weeks due to preterm labor, twins, and gestational diabetes, was coincidentally also a nurse. She made a list describing her good days and bad days and how to handle them:

Good days: feeling well, minimal contractions, in a routine with bedrest, productive, working on projects, thinking positive thoughts, planning baby's room, picking names, accepting and laughing about the situation.

On these days one should: remember them, they will return, cherish them, mark them on your calendar, stay busy, and feel productive.

Bad Days: many contractions, feeling blue, unproductive, scared, nervous, worrying if baby is all right, concerned about labor, hospitalization, afraid of baby dying, anxious about strain on you and your husband.

On these days one could: relax, if possible; pray, allow time to think, don't feel guilty about being nonproductive, do only the essentials - eat, drink, nap, take medicine, invite positive-minded friends and family, if you like or ask not to be disturbed, call your doctor with any medical questions, be well-informed, but don't diagnose yourself, ask to listen to the baby's heartbeat, talk to another mother on bedrest or a "graduate", cry, vent your feelings - talk with Dad, he may have similar feelings but tries to stay strong for you, remember this situation is temporary, daydream about things you will do with the new baby, talk, sing, or read to the baby, feel your abdomen, and feel the new life - the kicks and movements are very reassuring, call your minister, request a visit, call a therapist for counseling.

It is especially important to acknowledge and share how you are feeling. You have lost that ideal "normal" pregnancy which appears to come so easily to most every other mother. The feelings you have about this are normal. It is not uncommon to feel angry, disappointed, cheated, afraid, sad, lonely, resentful, hopeless, or discouraged. Sharing these feelings with loved ones and professionals can ease the burden.

Talk to your partner, to your parents, to your doctor, to your nurse, to your close friends, to your minister. If you are in the hospital, request to see the social worker. He or she can be of assistance in directing your concerns to appropriate resources, and in dealing with your emotions. Many hospitals now have referral lines for mothers on bedrest to contact other women in similar situations. Ask your nurse for the names and telephone extension of other mothers in the high risk unit. Visit and share by phone at least. One word of caution: Don't compare your pregnancy with that of any other woman. Each and every pregnancy is unique. Each woman's situation history, and physical status is different. Don't assume that since an acquaintance had preterm labor similar to yours that the rest of your pregnancy will be just like hers. The course of your pregnancy is dependent upon your situation, your history, your physical well-being, your therapies. There are too many variables to allow a prediction based on another's pregnancy. Every mother, high-risk or not, has an unparalleled story of the miraculous birth of her child.

You CAN have a semi-normal pregnancy ... but you WILL have to work for it.

Important Telephone Numbers

Beauty consultant (Avon, Mary Kay)

_____

Hair stylist (hospital/in-home)

_____

Library

_____

Bookstore

_____

Video store (delivery)

_____

Food (delivery)

_____

Minister

_____

Social Worker

_____

Therapist

_____

Mothers on bedrest referral line

_____

Other mothers on bedrest

_____

Offers of Assistance

Name	Phone number	Offered to:

III. "HOW IS THE BABY?"

How do you know your baby is okay? How can you tell if all this bedrest is really worth enduring? There is an array of tests which can answer these questions in a variety of ways. Collectively, this is known as antenatal testing. This simply means testing done before (ante) birth (natal). The range varies in simplicity, technology, risk, reliability, and results.

Not every high risk baby requires every antenatal test. Some babies will need only two or three of the least risky evaluations. For each of the most common tests, I will give a brief description of the methods used, the risk involved, and the results obtained. Be sure to ask your obstetrician for specifics concerning any tests he orders for your baby.

Also, it helps to remember that your baby is growing and developing constantly. New cells are forming every second. Check your baby's growth and chart it each week using the chart at the end of this chapter. Read any pamphlets you can find that describe fetal development. You might ask a friend to pick up a library book on the subject.

The earliest photographs of high risk babies are not the traditional pictures taken in the nursery a few hours or days after birth. They are not even found in videotaped deliveries. They are taken early in pregnancy by means of sonography. In preparation for an ultrasound exam, the mother is placed on her back on an examination table. Conductive lubricating jelly is then spread all over her abdomen. The technician sends high frequency sound waves, not electricity nor radiation, through the mother's belly toward her uterus and baby. The echo from those waves is recorded by the transducer, the instrument held by the technician, and is converted into an image on a screen. The mother will be requested to change position as needed to obtain a clear picture of certain parts of the baby's body. Copies of that image can become the first photo in your baby's record book.

More importantly, the pictures obtained can give your doctor information concerning your baby's well-being. Sonography can give required details about the number of fetuses, fetal position, fetal maturity, fetal growth, congenital abnormalities, placental position, and amniotic fluid volume. It is also used to assist in amniocentesis. Sonos can be performed at any time during pregnancy. An ultrasound produces no risk to you or to your baby.

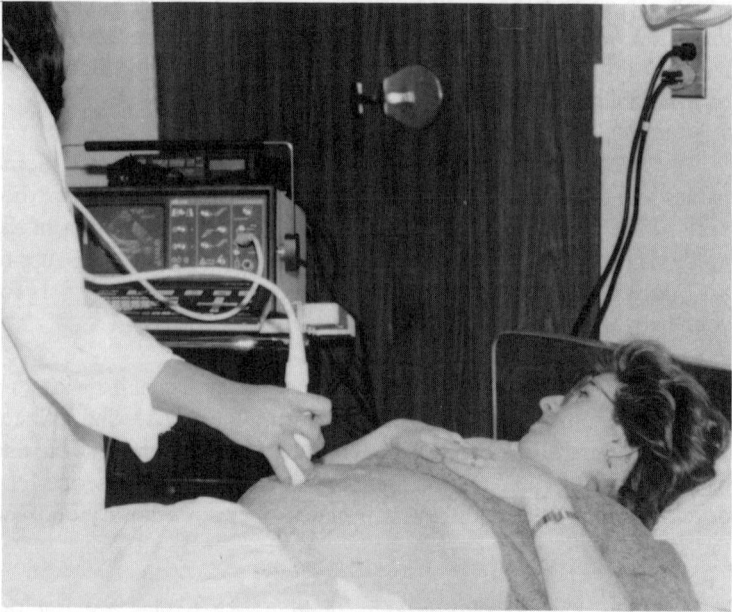

Sonogram in Progress.

At nine to twelve weeks, your baby's heart beat can be detected. The <u>fetal heart rate</u> can be heard by use of either a fetoscope or a doppler. The fetoscope is an odd-looking stethoscope which the obstetrician or nurse places on his head then presses to the mother's belly. A doppler is a small hand-held type of ultrasound instrument which amplifies the heart beat. The doppler lubricated with conductive jelly is placed on the mother's abdomen. The heartbeat is heard either through an attached stethoscope or a small portable amplifier. Again, there is no risk to either mother or baby.

The fetal heart rate is much faster than an adult's pulse. The normal range is 120-160 beats per minute. A decreased rate may indicate fetal distress. An increased rate may be the effect of medication (especially terbutaline and ritodrine), or congenital heart malformation. Any abnormal value is assessed by further testing.

At approximately 15 weeks, the baby's movements may be felt by the mother. Some mothers say the baby moves constantly while others say they hardly notice the movements during active parts of the day. Usually the baby is active after meals and, of course, at bedtime.

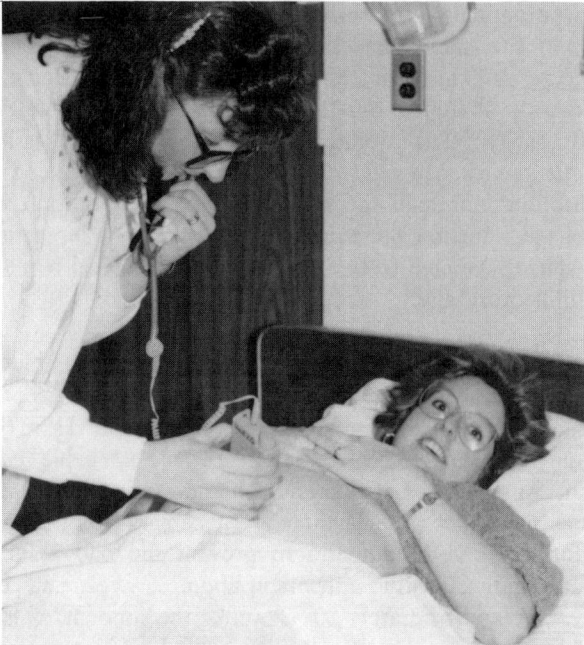

The Nurse Checks the Baby's heartbeat with a doppler.

Fetal activity can be an indicator of the baby's well-being. Each time you speak with your doctor or nurse, she may ask you if the baby has been active. You may be asked to keep a written record of the baby's movements. This record is called a fetal activity chart. You will be asked to lie on your left side for an hour after each meal and again at bedtime. During this time you should count the number of times the baby moves and write this number on a sheet of paper. If the baby moves more than five times or moves constantly during this time, you do not have to keep counting. It is enough to note that the baby was very active. If, however, the baby moves only five times or less, you should notify the nurse or doctor immediately. This may indicate that the baby is in distress. Fetal movement may also be slow due to medication. When you start any new medicine you should ask if it will affect the baby's activity, so you will not be alarmed unnecessarily. A fetal activity chart is provided at the end of this chapter.

The development of the baby's lungs is the most essential factor in determining how well the baby might fare if born prematurely. Lung development can be assessed before the baby is born by examination of the amniotic fluid. Amniotic fluid, the "water" in the sac which holds the baby, can be obtained by amniocentesis. This procedure involves inserting a needle through the mother's abdomen and the wall of the uterus and into the amniotic cavity. The mother's belly is first numbed with a local anesthetic, but she can still feel pressure of the needle being inserted. Complications, although uncommon, can include: abortion, maternal hemorrhage, infection, puncture wounds in the baby, laceration of the baby's spleen, damage to the placental and umbilical blood vessels, and fetal hemorrhage.[1]

The amniotic fluid analysis can reveal blood type incompatibilities (Rh factor), chromosomal disorders, some birth defects, the sex of the baby, as well as the L/S (lecithin/ sphingomyelin) ratio. The L/S ratio is the most reliable test for the baby's lung maturity. Lecithin and sphingomyelin are two chemicals known as surfactants. Surfactants are necessary to open the baby's lungs for the first breath and to prevent the baby's lungs from collapsing again. Lecithin appears at about 26 weeks and increases steadily. At approximately 30-32 weeks the amount of lecithin is usually 1.2 times greater than the amount of sphingomyelin. At 35 weeks, the ratio is 2:1.[2] While a ratio of 2.0 indicates that the lungs are definitely mature, a lower ratio does not necessarily mean that the baby will not survive. Your doctor can best tell you what your results mean for you and your baby.

It was helpful for me to know that preterm labor actually speeded the process of lung development. It seems that the stress placed on the baby causes increased steroid release which results in the development of surfactant. It was reassuring to know that some stress was actually helping the baby to prepare for the possibility of an early delivery.

Electronic fetal monitoring (EFM) is used to check the baby's heart rate, the mother's contractions, and the baby's reaction to the contractions. Internal monitoring is done by placing a tube through the vagina and cervix to record pressure changes caused by contractions and by placing a metal electrode onto the baby's scalp to monitor the baby's heartbeat. To use an internal monitor, the membranes must have ruptured and the cervix must be dilated.

External monitoring is done by placing two belts around the mother's belly. The first holds a doppler which picks up the baby's heartbeat and converts it into both an audible beat and a printed graph of the heart rate. The second belt holds a tocodynamometer, or toco, which is a plastic meter that can sense the tightening of contractions and convert it into a printed graph of the length and frequency of contractions. External monitoring can be done anytime after the heartbeat can be heard with a doppler and does not require ruptured membranes or a dilated cervix since it is not invasive. External monitors are used for high risk mothers to check on the presence and frequency of contractions. Sometimes you may not be aware of minor contractions which may indicate preterm labor. External monitors also help to record the reaction of the baby's heart to the baby's movements and to contractions. The baby's heart rate should increase when the baby moves and during contractions, just as your heart rate increases when you exercise or are under stress.

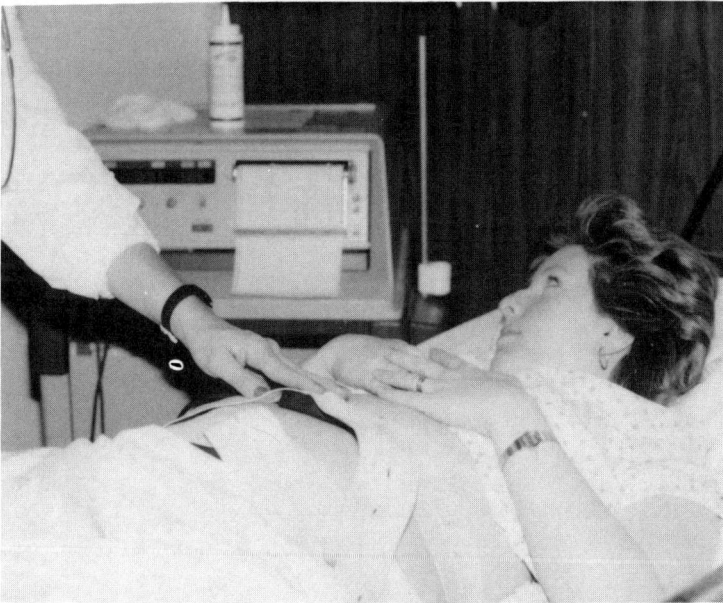

External Fetal Monitor.

External monitoring done for twenty to forty minutes is known as a non-stress test. A reactive test indicates a normal healthy baby with a good chance of survival. A non-reactive test indicates some abnormality or possible fetal distress. A non-reactive NST is usually followed by a stress test, also known as a contraction stress test (CST) or oxytocin challenge test (OCT). In an OCT, contractions are stimulated by giving a medication called oxytocin to the mother through an IV. Again, the reaction of the baby's heart rate to the contraction is monitored. A negative test indicates that the baby is not in distress. A positive test indicates that the baby may be in distress and may not tolerate labor well. This test is usually not done prior to 28 weeks because it may start the labor process. You should know that having this test done means being prepared to deliver if the test is positive.

A biophysical profile (BPP) utilizes electronic fetal monitoring in conjunction with sonography to assess your baby. It results in a score between 0 and 10, with 10 indicating that the baby is doing well. Any score less than 6 would alert the doctor to possible fetal distress. BPP's may be ordered on a regular schedule.

My Antenatal Tests

My first sonogram was done on (date)_____

  It showed:_____

_____

_____

Other sonograms:

  <u>Date</u>   <u>Results</u>

_____

_____

_____

_____

_____

_____

The first time I heard the baby's heartbeat was:_____

_____

  The rate was:_____ beats per minute.

Other times I heard the baby's heartbeat:

		Heart rate
<u>Date</u>	<u># weeks</u>	<u>(# beats per minute)</u>
_____	10	_____
_____	11	_____
_____	12	_____
_____	13	_____
_____	14	_____
_____	15	_____
_____	16	_____
_____	17	_____
_____	18	_____

Date	# weeks	Heart rate (# beats per minute)
	19	
	20	
	21	
	22	
	23	
	24	
	25	
	26	
	27	
	28	
	29	
	30	
	31	
	32	
	33	
	34	
	35	
	36	
	37	
	38	
	39	
	40	

My Antenatal Tests

My first amniocentesis was done on (date):_____

The results:_____

_____

_____

Other amniocenteses:

<u>Date</u>   <u>Results</u>

_____

_____

_____

_____

My first time on the electronic fetal monitor was (date):

_____

The baby's heart rate was (# beats per minute):_____

Contractions:_____

Other times on the monitor:

<u>Date</u> <u>Heart rate</u> <u>Contractions?</u>

_____

_____

_____

_____

_____

_____

_____

_____

_____

Fetal Activity Chart

Date	Time	# of Movements	Date	Time	# of Movements

IV. "BUT ... WHAT ABOUT MY OTHER CHILDREN?"

"It's eleven p.m. Do you know where your children are?" When I was a teenager, I used to chuckle at this introduction to the late news. Now that I'm a parent, it doesn't seem so funny. When I was in the hospital on bedrest, a more urgent question was, "Who can we find to watch the boys tomorrow?" My mom, my sisters, and my brother, all worked full-time during the day. So, while they all pitched in to help in the evenings and on the weekends, we still needed someone who could watch three-year-old Matthew and eighteen-month old Christopher on weekdays while Michael worked. Fortunately, we discovered we had many able-bodied volunteers. And so do you!

If you have time to read this, I assume you found someone to care for your child(ren) while you saw the doctor and were told to be on bedrest, whether at home or in the hospital. The more common problem is how to manage childcare when you are unsure of how long you will need it. Unless you have been told otherwise, assume you will be on bedrest until delivery, hopefully near your due date. Plan accordingly. I used my calendar to decide when I needed childcare and to keep track of who would watch the boys and where. If you have more than one place or person for your child, I suggest you do the same. You can do that from bed! Keep your phone, phone book, calendar, and pencil ready. Notice I said pencil. Be sure it has an eraser. Plans change - people get sick, their children get the chicken pox, friends have other plans. You may need to make alternate arrangements more than once. Keep a list of anyone who offers to help with your children, even if you're not sure he/she is the ideal baby-sitter. You might get desperate enough to settle for less than an ideal situation.

There was a time, when I was 28 weeks pregnant and in the hospital on bedrest, when all my volunteers were either busy, or sick, or had sick children. I didn't know where to turn. Michael had just started a new job. He had already taken several unearned days off. His boss was more than reasonable about our circumstances, but Michael couldn't stay home any more than absolutely necessary. When I mentioned this to my pastor he reminded me that some church members whom I didn't even know had offered to look after the boys. Reluctantly, I called one of these volunteers. An entry in my journal tells the rest of the story:

"I was very anxious about the boys on Wednesday without cause. They stayed with Jean Harberts and her boys, Kyle and Zachary. I knew Jean only as the Mom of Zachary, who was in St. Michael's nursery with Christopher. But I needn't have worried - Kyle and Matthew were instant friends. 'He has trains and a little baby brother - just like me!' (Kyle is also 3 1/2 years old, Zach is one year old.)"

In your search for childcare, it's best to start with the people with whom your children are most familiar. So, if Grandmom, PopPop, or other close relatives are willing and able, pick up their offers. You might also ask neighbors, friends, and parents of your children's friends. Don't forget to inquire at your church office for possible volunteers!

Volunteers are a great boon to the budget, especially if your income is decreased while you are on bedrest. However, if your child was in a day care situation - with a baby-sitter, a day care home, or a day care center - and you can afford to continue this routine, it might be best to do so.

If you do not have an established day care arrangement and you have run out of volunteers, you may be able to find a sitter to employ either at your house or at the sitter's home. Ask friends, relatives, coworkers, and the church office for recommendations. Nearby community colleges or universities may have job placement offices which can be helpful. The Department of Social Services maintains a list of licensed day care providers which they can make available to you. Mothers of Multiples clubs sometimes have support services and/or child care information. A call to your local Girl Scout troop may result in referrals of Scouts interested in earning child care badges. (They might also want to meet requirements for cooking or community service badges.) Your local library may have information on before and after school care, summer camps, vacation Bible schools, licensed day care providers, nannies, and au pair services.

Even ideal childcare arrangements do not prevent the emotional trauma which results from your abrupt, unexplained absence. When I had been in the hospital for two weeks, Matthew, my three-year-old began to tell my husband, "I'll never see Mom again." I was devastated! That night I wrote: "It's been such a long time for him that I've not been home. I'm sure he's confused, maybe angry that I 'left him.' I know that he knows something about your coming and that we have to wait 'til it's safe. I'm not sure how much to make of this or quite what, if anything, I should do. Maybe I'll talk with Dr. Zern tomorrow. She, being a mom and an M.D. might have some insight."

Though I didn't speak to my OB the next day, I did gain some good advice from my pediatrician. He reassured me that Matthew's behavior was normal; apathetic, withdrawn, or abusive behavior, however, may be cause for concern. He also reminded me that when I did go home that I would be adding insult to injury by bringing the baby who would require much of my time and attention. He suggested that we bring a gift for him from the baby at that time.

On Matthew's first visit to the hospital I had explained to him why I was there, what all the equipment did, how the baby was doing, and when I expected to be home. From his statement, I realized that constant reinforcement of this information and more was needed. From other Moms, I have discovered that each child will require different types and amount of information depending on the child's age and personality. All children should be allowed to visit and should be reassured that Mom will be coming home. Don't promise anything you can't deliver. (Pardon the pun.) You might spend one visit making a calendar, marking the due date and counting down the days. Make a duplicate - one for your room and one for your child's room.

Explain your environment in terms your children will understand. Allow them to experiment with those things which are safe. My sons delighted in being in charge of the console which controlled the TV and the lights in the room. Do not allow them to readjust the bed if you are required to stay in a certain position. And, please, do not allow them to use the intercom unless you need to call the nurse. Unnecessary use of the intercom not only annoys the ward clerk and nurses, but also prevents other patients from obtaining assistance.

Plan your visits. Make them as frequent as possible, but keep them short. You may be surprised how tired you are after they leave. Prepare for visits by having supplies brought in. These supplies may include: scrap paper, construction paper, crayons, pencils, markers, scissors, glue, books, small toys, board games, snacks, and more. You might keep it all in a small cardboard or plastic box just for them. They'll look forward to taking it out when they come. Update your calendar each time they stop in. Use markers or stickers to count down the days. Have your children indicate special days and events to come with their own drawings. Put artwork and/or school papers on exhibit. Be sure to include family pictures. Allow your child to take pictures of you that he might keep at home. A Polaroid camera works best for this.

Share with your child any information you have about the baby. Tell him how much the baby has grown. Listen to the baby's heartbeat together. Let him feel the baby kick and move. Look at pictures of fetal development at each stage. Talk about how your child also grew like this, and is continuing to grow. Ask someone to bring your child's baby album to share.

End each visit by planning the next one. When will it be? What will you do? Again, mark it on the calendar. Listen to your child's fears and repeat them to him. Answer all questions truthfully, without smothering your child in details. Explain to him or her that plans might change, but be sure to give reassurance of your love.

After visits, try to arrange for someone to be available at home with whom your child can talk openly about his feelings and his perspective of the situation. This person could be Dad or Grandmom or a neighbor or a teacher. Children quickly perceive when all is not well and need to vent their feelings in a safe environment. They need to be reassured that it is okay to have these feelings and may need direction in channeling their reactions.

You, too, need to vent your feelings. If you don't have a diary or journal, this may be the perfect time to start one. More than once you may need to speak openly and aloud (perhaps very loud) about your predicament. You may not want to burden your husband or other family members who are taking on some of your responsibilities. Perhaps you have a friend or relative who is a good listener. Sometimes it helps to talk to someone in a more objective, detached position or someone with more professional health knowledge. In this case, your nurse, obstetrician, pediatrician, minister, rabbi, or social worker may be a good resource. On short notice, God is always waiting and available. Prayer, with or without tears, was always effective for me.

Home monitoring is now a popular option for patients without previa or PROM. An electronic fetal monitor is delivered to your home. You are taught to apply the doppler and tocodynamometer and to call a central monitoring office. Qualified RN's assess your computerized readout and notify you and your doctor of any indication for change in your therapy.

Patrick is now three years old. Christopher, who was eighteen months old during my hospitalization, remembers only family stories and pictures of that time. In addition, Matthew who was then 3 1/2 years old recalls vaguely that I spent "a little while" in the hospital "because Patrick wanted to be born too early." Obviously, my boys have all survived with no emotional scars. What seems like an imminent emotional tragedy will most likely be forgotten by your baby's first birthday.

V. "HOW WILL I PAY FOR ALL OF THIS?"

You may know why you are on bedrest, how you will manage, how the baby is doing and how your other children are, but do you know how much this will cost or how you will pay for it? I can't offer to foot the bill, but I can tell you it's better to be prepared if you can. There are certain steps you can and should take as soon as you can. There are other actions which have to wait until after delivery.

Right now, you should call your health insurance provider. Ask for the name and title of the person taking your call. Be sure to have ready your policy identification number, the name of the person insured, and the group number if you have one. Describe your current situation and any anticipated changes. If you are at home, but expect to be hospitalized at some point, tell them now.

Ask for all the details related to your coverage. What services are covered? If applicable, ask about home monitoring, hospitalization for high risk pregnancy, medications, terbutaline pump (inpatient or at home), home health nurses and/or aides. What is the deductible, the copayment, the maximum out-of pocket expenses? How and when should charges be submitted? If possible, have all this information sent to you in writing. You may need this documentation.

Next, call your hospital billing office. You may be referred to the admitting office, the obstetrics admitting office, or the hospital social worker. Get the name and title of the person or persons who give you any information. If you are in the hospital, you may have already been contacted, or will be shortly. If you are at home, but expect to be hospitalized prior to delivery, it may be helpful for you to call now. Even mothers with uncomplicated pregnancies are now contacted well before their due date by the hospital billing office. Many hospitals now request your insurance information with registration so they may obtain a predetermination of benefits from your provider. This predetermination will tell the hospital (and you) exactly what services are covered, the amount which is covered, and what amount is your responsibility. Based on this information, the hospital may require a partial or full prepayment of your deductible, co-payments, and uncovered services. Again, ask that all this information be sent to you in writing.

61

Armed with all this data, <u>enlist the support of your hospital social worker.</u> She knows the bureaucracy and the resources. She can answer most of your questions. She is your financial (and emotional) advocate. The hospital wants her to help you find a way to pay the bill. Thus, they cooperate with her.

A payment plan may be offered by the hospital to alleviate a large one-time charge. If the bill is still overwhelming, there are alternatives. Most hospitals have charity funds available to assist with hardship cases. This may be through the hospital auxiliary or community grants.

You may qualify for Medical Assistance in one of several ways. You may be eligible for all your medical, hospital, and medication expenses to be paid. Or, you may qualify for a one-time payment from Medical Assistance for catastrophic bills. This depends on your income, the number of dependent children, the length of your hospital stay, and the size of your bill. Call your local Medical Assistance office or ask your social worker about this resource.

Your social worker may be helpful in other areas, as well. She may be able to assist in child-care resources or arrangements. She may be able to help your family get a parking pass for frequent visits if your stay is expected to be lengthy or undetermined. Parking fees can mount quickly. Don't let this isolate you from your family.

You might also <u>solicit the assistance of your obstetrician.</u> My doctor wrote several letters to my insurance company to explain my situation and the reasons for my hospitalization. She told me that she made it very clear that the cost of my care on a high-risk antepartal unit was much less expensive than the care of a premature baby in the NICU (neonatal intensive care unit). They were apparently convinced. Fortunately, the amount of the hospital bill which we were required to pay was manageable.

After you deliver, are discharged, and are enjoying your newborn, the bills will continue to come in the mail. These may include charges for radiology, anesthesiology, your hospital stay, your baby's hospital stay and care, and NICU services. Call your hospital, your social worker, and the providers of these services if you have any questions, or if you have trouble paying any of the bills. Apply for any financial aid you need. Remember to check with the hospital, the hospital auxiliary, Medical Assistance, your church, and local community agencies.

The hospital social worker may be aware of even more local resources. Be sure to contact her with any questions.

Financial Information

Insurance information

Health insurance provider: _____

   Name of insured:_____

   Group number:_____

   Identification number:_____

   Address: _____

   _____

   Phone number: _____

   Name and title of person(s) giving information: _____

   _____

Secondary provider (if any):_____

   Name of insured:_____

   Group number:_____

   Identification number:_____

   Address:_____

   _____

   _____

   Phone number:_____

   Name and Title of person(s) giving information:_____

   _____

   _____

   _____

Hospital Billing Office

   Phone number:_____

   Name and Title of person(s) giving information:_____

      _____

      _____

      _____

Hospital Social Worker

   Name and Title:_____

      _____

   Phone number: _____

Medical Assistance

   Name and Title of person(s) giving information:_____

      _____

      _____

   Phone number:_____

VI. "WHAT DO I TELL MY BOSS?"

You may or may not have previously informed your employer of your pregnancy and/or of your maternity leave plans. In either case, now is the time for a phone call to your boss. Do not leave your supervisor guessing as to your whereabouts. Tell him/her that you are pregnant and are experiencing some difficulties. You do not need to share all the details.

You should call the Personnel office immediately and notify them of your need for a short term disability leave. High risk pregnancy requiring bedrest is not considered an illness. You may not need or want to use sick leave. You are not eligible for maternity leave until you have delivered.

Inquire about your company's temporary disability policy and follow it. Use your employee handbook, if you have one, to determine procedures to be followed, forms to be filed, persons to be notified. Notify them by phone and follow up with a letter which includes all the details which were discussed. Most employers will require a letter from your doctor. Determine the necessary information which must be included and relay this to your doctor's office. Or, write the letter for your doctor to sign.

If you have any questions about your leave status, call your personnel office, or labor union. Your social worker may also be of assistance in sorting out any problems with your employer. You may also wish to contact the Department of Labor, Human Relations Commission, or Office of Public Affairs for clarification of relevant federal, state, and/or local regulations.

Keep your immediate supervisor updated on your status. When it is convenient, call your boss to discuss your work just prior to bedrest so your coworkers can pick up where you left off. Keep up with the progress of any projects in which you were involved.

If you wish to work from bed, work out the details. Make arrangements for delivery of necessary paperwork or materials. Put all agreements in writing and send a copy to your boss, to payroll, and to personnel. Don't try to accomplish everything you did at the office. Plan rest periods and anticipate the possibility of the need for unplanned rest periods.

Whether and how you will be paid during your leave of absence will be determined by your employer, union, and local regulations. Your status within the company should be determined by company policy, written or unwritten. If you are aware of a similar circumstance in which an employee was paid during a temporary leave, then you, too, should be eligible for pay during this leave. If, in a similar situation, an employee's position and/or status was retained, then your position should also be retained. Call the Department of Labor if you need details or more information.

Be honest with your boss. Tell him/her that you do not know if, or when you will be able to return to work. Again, keep your supervisor up to date concerning your work status. Call in on a regular basis, even if you do not have any new information. Do inform them of the date of your delivery. This is when maternity leave begins. Barring any unforeseen complications, this is when you become a "normal" mom.

Work-related Phone Numbers

Immediate Supervisor:_____

_____

Personnel Office:_____

_____

Labor Union:_____

_____

VII. "IT TAKES TWO!"

Okay ... where is he? It took two of you to get into this situation. Don't exclude Dad now! If he's not in shock or in hiding, he's probably been beside you most, if not all, of the time since you discovered you are a high risk mom. If he hasn't been involved, now is the time to include him.

I don't need to tell you that this is a very stressful time in your relationship. Don't forget that there is a relationship! Under stress, it becomes extremely important that you communicate clearly and regularly. All the good and bad in the relationship tends to be emphasized under duress.

Whenever possible, Dad should be included. This does not mean that he must take off work for every test and/or doctor's appointment. He should, however, be kept aware of appointments, doctor's advice, test results, changes in your physical and emotional states, and the need for decisions.

If Dad does not accompany you to appointments, you should discuss them before and after they occur. Share your concerns, questions, and feelings. Ask about his concerns, questions and feelings. Involve him in all decision-making processes. The results of these decisions affect him as well as you.

Listen! Listen, listen, and then listen again. Pay attention to nonverbal cues, especially if he is the strong, silent type.

Plan date nights - at home or in the hospital. Order takeout food delivered to your room. Rent a video or a new video game. Play a board or card game. Set aside time to be together without dwelling on the obvious difficulties.

Don't expect him to be with you always. He has to work, get the laundry done, fix meals, maintain the house, take care of the older child(ren), prepare home for the new baby, keep in touch with friends and family, and rest. He needs private time, as usual, especially considering the stress he's under.

There were several times while I was hospitalized that I thought that delivery may be imminent. I felt I should call Michael but did not wish to alarm him unnecessarily. He had just recently started a new job and, thus, had not accumulated vacation time. Also, I had to consider who would care for our two sons at two a.m. If it was a reasonable time of day, I called him to be on standby. In the middle of the night, I asked the Delivery Room nurse to call him if the situation became serious. He never did need to come in unexpectedly.

Help him in whatever way you can from bed. Schedule baby-sitting/day care arrangements by phone. Keep up the household paperwork, pay the bills, call the plumber, order takeout food, and accept and schedule any and all offers of help (lawn-mowing, meals, childcare, housework, laundry). Give him a back rub. Schedule and encourage time for him to play and to rest.

Dad! Are you listening? This is for you, too. Mom needs your help in more ways than may be apparent. Listen to her, encourage her to share her concerns and feelings. Be there for her to hold your hand or cry on your shoulder.

Include her in the real world. Don't keep everyday events, decisions, and/or problems from her. She wants to know what's happening "out there". She doesn't want to know about every squabble between siblings, but inform her of any emotional changes they may have. Keep her up to date, as you usually would, about your work, your friends, and your family. Let her be as active in your family life as possible.

Attempt to keep your home as orderly as possible. Be realistic, but try to do those things which you know are of special concern to your wife. Graciously accept all offers of help. This is not the time to be macho - you can not do it all alone. Rely on Mom for phone contacts, scheduling of child care, anything she is allowed to do. When an offer is made, make note of it for future reference. You may not need it immediately, but it may be the perfect solution to a future problem.

Plan special times for the two of you, for each of your children with you and with her, separately and together.

Be flexible. Physically, things could change from minute to minute. Plans may need to be changed at any time. Be alert to her emotions. Ask when she would like time alone, when she would like to see the children, when she desires visitors. Keep open the lines of communication.

Alert your boss to the situation. Prepare arrangements at work in case you need to leave quickly to be with Mom. Decrease overtime hours, if possible. Try to decrease any work-related stress - you have enough at home.

There are, in some areas, not only support groups (or hotlines, or networks) for mothers on bedrest, but also resources for high risk dads. Ask your doctor, nurse, social worker, or hospital about the availability of such resources in your area. Enlist the aid of the hospital parent education office. Talking to fathers who have experienced or are experiencing a high risk pregnancy can be invaluable. Also, Dad, be sure to read the rest of this book!

VIII. "READY FOR DELIVERY?"

"READY?! I'm not ready for any of this! I planned a normal pregnancy and delivery! You know the kind ... with maternity clothes, baby showers, special privileges, childbirth classes, fixing up the baby's room, buying cute little outfits. How can I plan anything now?!" This is certainly how I felt when asked what type of delivery I was planning. I had lost all control of my future. This was my third child. I should have been a veteran by this point. Yet, here I was, having had in my lifetime only one class in childbirth education. I had never delivered according to the book. After seven years of unsuccessfully attempting to get and stay pregnant, we adopted Matthew. Even he was born three weeks early and had complications. We had arranged legal custody from birth and were on hand for delivery. However, our plans for taking him home after 24 hours were waylaid due to jaundice, pneumonia, and an infection of his umbilical cord. His discharge was delayed for eight days.

Christopher made an early surprise entry at 31 weeks, just days after our first, and only, childbirth class. After a sudden, bloody rupture of membranes, I started contracting but never dilated. After 12 hours of labor a caesarean section was performed. He was sent to a regional neonatal intensive care unit at another hospital. I didn't see him for four days. He remained in the NICU for a month. Due to a digestive disorder, he was placed on an apnea monitor for almost a year. Before the monitor was gone, I realized I was pregnant again. We thought we had a chance at a normal, if caesarean, delivery.

This time, we started by planning for the worst and hoping for the best. We searched for an obstetrician with some expertise in caring for high risk mothers. Unfortunately, we needed that expertise sooner than expected. Early dilation required a cervical suture at 19 weeks. This was my introduction to bedrest. I was at home on bedrest for seven weeks, until the contractions began. We rushed to the hospital expecting to lose this baby. However, by the next morning the contractions were under control and I was introduced to strict bedrest in the high risk obstetrical unit. Any further "planning" for delivery was to be done from this horizontal position. Patrick was born vaginally at 37 1/2 weeks with no complications. Though our plans were disheveled, the delivery was wonderful!

I had lost all control of my future, but I was determined to use my "rest" period wisely. You may be surprised at how much you can do from your bed!

You can prepare yourself and your husband by learning all you can about this baby. Books and videotapes about your baby's growth and development, about baby care and feeding, and about safety and discipline are available from a variety of sources. The public library, bookstores, video stores, the hospital library, the health department, the hospital gift shop, the hospital parent education office, your doctor, and your nurse will each have some of this information for you. Local branches of La Leche League, and the Childbirth Education Association can help you learn about breast-feeding. You do have time to learn!

You and your husband can also prepare for the actual delivery. First, be prepared for nothing to go according to plan. Anything that does meet your expectations is then a plus.

Second, if you don't already know, find out what your options are. Ask your doctor if a caesarean delivery is best or if a vaginal delivery is possible. Each mother's circumstances are different and may change at any time. Be prepared for all options.

Third, contact your hospital's parent education office, your doctor, or the local Childbirth Education Association office concerning childbirth preparation classes. You may not be able to attend the regular classes, but there may be alternatives. Some hospitals offer at-home or in-hospital tutoring. They will arrange to bring all the materials to your bedside at a time convenient for you and your husband and/or labor coach. Videos of actual classes may be available. Special classes are usually offered for caesarean sections and for breast-feeding. Refresher courses are also available for those who have delivered previously.

Most childbirth preparation classes include a tour of the labor and delivery suite and of the post-partum units of the hospital. So, where does that leave you? (Other than in bed, of course). Well, actually you have several alternatives. If it is safe for you and your baby, your doctor may allow you to physically take the tour. This is one time when being on bedrest in the hospital is an advantage. You may be able to arrange a private tour with your nurse. A wheelchair or stretcher may be your mode of transportation. Older children may also enjoy this outing. However, if you must remain on strict bedrest, you can use the VCR again. If no ready-made tape of the tour is available, arrange for one to be made. Your husband or coach could tape his/her tour with your camera or with one on loan from the hospital, a friend, or a video store. Even without a camera, your husband can give you at least a complete description. You may be able to arrange to talk with a nurse from the delivery suite either in person or on the phone. She could explain routines and answer your questions.

Fourth, arrange a similar tour of the Neonatal Intensive Care Unit (NICU). Even if you make it to term, complications could require your baby to be observed in the NICU. It is much easier to look at the NICU when your baby is not in it. Even with no emotional ties, the equipment and the environment can be overwhelming. It will be very warm because the premature babies cannot maintain an even body temperature. It will be crowded due to all the equipment required. And, it will be noisy due to the machinery and the alarms. Take the time to ask any questions which come to mind. Again, if you cannot physically tour the NICU, arrange for a NICU nurse to visit or call. In some hospitals the staff neonatalogist (doctor who specializes in premature and newborn care) will visit high risk mothers who are in the hospital. If the hospital at which you plan to deliver does not have a NICU, ask where your baby might be sent and contact that NICU for information.

Finally, act like normal parents and get ready for that baby. He/she will need a name, diapers, clothes, a place to sleep, and a thousand other things. So you better get started.

Interviewing a pediatrician is of primary importance. "But ...", I hear you say, "I'm on bedrest, remember!" Believe me, it's not easy to forget. However, this is no excuse for neglecting your duty. You can call your hospital for physician referrals. Most hospitals will give you a list of pediatricians in your area, along with addresses and, most importantly, their phone numbers. Ask friends, family, neighbors, day-care providers, librarians, your nurses, and your obstetrician for their recommendations.

Call those doctors who appeal to you. Ask the receptionist to have the doctor call you at a convenient time to discuss his practice. Check his hours, location, on-call schedule, telephone hours, emergency contact procedure, and basic child care philosophy. Perhaps your husband, or friend, or a family member could videotape a tour of his office. If you are on bedrest in a hospital at which he has privileges, ask if he might stop to see you the next time he is there to see patients. This may give you an indication of his flexibility.

Once you have made a decision, be sure to record your pediatrician's name and phone number in a convenient place. Space is provided at the end of this chapter. Also, notify your obstetrician, your nurse, and the hospital where you plan to deliver. This will increase the chances of your pediatrician being notified promptly of delivery.

Have you chosen your baby's name? Volumes of names are available from the library and bookstores. Pharmaceutical companies distribute lists of names to obstetricians, hospitals and clinics. And, no doubt, your friends and relatives will have a few suggestions. Try them out. A friend of mine tried screaming names to hear how she would sound when trying to get the attention of her toddler-to-be. Quietly repeating the full name and anticipated nicknames is more traditional.

What type of diapers will you use? Once you decide whether you will use cloth or disposable, you can arrange to have them delivered to your home. Ask a friend to shop for you, or have a case sent by a department store. You can prearrange diaper service by phone. You have time to comparison shop either way.

You can also choose birth announcements. Parent and family magazines have quite a few ads for catalogs of cards. Stationers may send you samples. Local card stores may agree to send some home with a friend for your approval. The envelopes can be addressed and stamped now, saving valuable time after the baby is born.

Clothes and accessories can be ordered by phone or by mail through a myriad of mail-order and department store catalogs. You can also order curtains, linens, even furniture. Just have someone else do all the measuring. Delivery of these items can be conveniently arranged, either before or after the baby is born.

If your due date is far enough away, you may have time to <u>direct</u> the preparation of the baby's room. You may not be able to paint or wallpaper, but you can certainly choose the colors and patterns.

There! I told you, you have plenty of preparation you can do from that bed. Now get started ... this bedrest won't last forever!

<u>La Leche League</u>

Local chapter phone number: _____

<u>Hospital:</u> _____

Address and phone number: _____

_____

_____

Parent education office: _____

Labor and delivery: _____

Neonatal Intensive Care: _____

Hospital library: _____

Gift shop: _____

<u>Childbirth Education Association</u>

Local office and phone number: _____

_____

_____

<u>Pediatrician</u>

Address: _____

_____

_____

Phone number: _____

IX. "I NEED A PROJECT!"

After twenty weeks of pregnancy bedrest, the most frequent question posed to me is "What did you do all that time?" Well, I did a little bit of everything possible from a horizontal position. I kept my sanity by keeping busy. At first, it was easy. At home, I updated our photo albums, the boy's baby books, our financial records, our address book, my recipe files, my coupon file, and the birthday calendar. Then I did our tax return and read a few novels. I completed some long-ago abandoned cross-stitch work. Then I got desperate and finished the entire pile of mending. By the time I was in the hospital on bedrest, there was little left to update. I began reading more novels, calling more friends (or the same ones more frequently), polishing and unpolishing my nails more than once a day, and increasingly watching too much TV by default. Soon, I found myself calling everyone I knew to tell them, "I need a project!"

I volunteered to do just about any type of paperwork or needlework. Quite a few people took up the offer. I cut out paper sheep for Sunday School, made banners for our Marriage Encounter group, framed some of my mother's cross-stitch pieces, addressed shower invitations, made shower favors, addressed wedding invitations, and even finished a friend's needlework project. In a moment of total boredom, I recalled a ceramic nativity set I had left unpainted in the attic for ten years. My husband brought in the pieces so I'd have a few more days' work to do. I was rarely longer than a few hours without a project.

I have listed below all the "projects" I can remember doing along with some suggestions from other high risk moms. It is by no means an exhaustive listing but merely a springboard for your imagination. Use this time to its full potential. Unfortunately, the time cannot be bottled for use six months after delivery!

Arts and Crafts

cross-stitch	wreaths
needlework	framing
ceramics	sew
dried flower arrangements	color
mend	paint

79

Children's Activities

crayons	photos
paints	puppets
play dough	polish nails
school work	tea parties
calendar	read/tell stories
talk about baby	board games

plan for big brother/sister role
computer games - Atari, Nintendo
plan activities for after delivery
have seasonal "events" - egg hunt, birthday party, Halloween
   costume parade, Christmas caroling, etc.

Date Night with Dad
   order out - pizza to gourmet
   movies - TV or VCR
   games - board, computer
   cards
   try a massage
   invite friends for dinner, snack, games, movies (order out or
      have Dad or friends fix food)

Entertain
   order out - breakfast, lunch, dinner, snack
   have a tea or coffee klatsch - make it pot luck
   celebrate a friend's birthday with a cake or ice cream

Games
   chess
   checkers
   backgammon
   cards
   crossword puzzles
   word searches
   mind games
   computer games - Atari, Nintendo
   board games - have you mastered Trivial Pursuit, or tried
      Scruples?

Health/Beauty
      give yourself a manicure
      have your hair cut, colored, or styled - some stylists will come to the house or even the hospital. Ask your nurse for a referral for an in-hospital stylist.
      have a friend or professional give you a pedicure
      give yourself a facial
      get a massage
      request a physical therapy consult for exercises you can do
      have a make-over party with a friend or two

Phone
      arrange childcare
      call schools, teachers to keep in touch
      make work arrangements
      call library for books (see Read)
      make insurance arrangements
      mail order - gifts, maternity clothes, diapers/diaper service, baby clothes, baby accessories, baby room decorations, birth announcements, etc.

Plan
      things to do after delivery
      write reminders, lists
      order travel brochures
      plan a trip or vacation - AAA will help

Read
      novels   magazines
      journals   newspapers
      Bible   Bible studies
      suggested topics - growth and development
            childbirth education
            infant care
            normal pregnancy
            high risk pregnancy
            parenting styles

Seasonal
      tax returns
      Christmas shopping (mail order)
      Christmas cards
      Easter egg hunt in your room

Seasonal (Continued)
    decorate room with seasonal theme
    plan garden, order seeds, plants, equipment

TV/VCR
    movies   soap operas
    news/talk shows   infant care tapes
    childbirth education tapes   sports specials
    tours of labor/delivery/NICU
    homemade tapes of school/home events, even routine
        happenings
    tapes of your church worship service

Update
    recipe files
    photo albums
    household finances
    birthday calendar
    phone/address book
    baby books for other children
    calendar
    car - preventive maintenance or major repairs. Have a
        friend take it to the garage for you - you won't need it for
        awhile.

Volunteer
    Church/place of worship - paperwork, cut, collate, fold, stuff
        and/or address envelopes, prepare Sunday school
        materials.
    School - prepare bulletin board materials, class materials,
        etc.
    invitations - offer to prepare, stuff, stamp, and address a
        friend's wedding/shower/party invitations

Work
    any desk work or paperwork which can be brought to you
    phone calls
    appointments - by phone or arrange for bedside
        appointments
    typing/word processing if you are allowed to sit up at all
    grade papers or prepare lesson plans, if you teach

Write

      journal/diary entries
      letters to out-of-town friends
      cards - birthday, thank you notes
      birth announcements - fill in your names, address envelopes
      family tree
      calendar
      letters to insurance company to document need for bedrest

Chapter I

[1] Elizabeth Stepp Gilbert and Judith Smith Harmon, High Risk Pregnancy and Delivery (St. Louis: The C.V. Mosby Co., 1986) 279

[2] Sheldon B. Korones, High Risk Newborn Infants: The Basis for Intensive Nursing Care (St. Louis: The C.V. Mosby Co., 1986) 34

[3] F. Gary Cunningham, M.D., Paul C. MacDonald, M.D., and Norman F. Gant, M.D., Williams Obstetrics (18th ed.; Norwalk, Conn.: Appleton and Lange, 1989) 676

[4] Cunningham, MacDonald, and Gant 712

[5] Gilbert and Harmon 233

[6] Susan R. Givens, "Update on Tocolytic Therapy in the Management of Preterm Labor," The Journal of Perinatal and Neonatal Nursing July 1988: 22

[7] Gilbert and Harmon 312

[8] Cunningham, MacDonald, and Gant 752

[9] Gilbert and Harmon 326

[10] Cunningham, MacDonald, and Gant 632

[11] M.C. Saunders, J. Dick, I. McL. Brown, K. McPherson, and I. Chalmers, "The Effects of Hospital Admission for Bedrest on the Duration of Twin Pregnancy: A Randomised Trial," The Lancet October 12, 1985: 793
Bela Komaromy and Lazlo Lampe, "The Value of Bedrest in Twin Pregnancies," International Journal of Gynecology and Obstetrics 15 (1977): 262
L.C. Gilstrap III, J.C. Hauth, G.D.V. Hankins, and A. Beck, "Twins: Prophylactic Hospitalization and Ward Rest at Early Gestational Age, Obstetrics and Gynecology 69.4 (April 1987): 578

Cunningham, MacDonald, and Gant 643

[12] Cunningham, MacDonald, and Gant 644

[13] Gilbert and Harmon 268
[14] Cunningham, MacDonald, and Gant 653-6

[15] Cunningham, MacDonald, and Gant 674
Gilbert and Harmon 276-8

[16] Cunningham, MacDonald, and Gant 277

[17] Cunningham, MacDonald, and Gant 673

[18] L.B. Curet and R.W. Olson, "Evaluation of a Program of Bedrest in the Treatment of Chronic Hypertension in Pregnancy," Obstetrics and Gynecology 53.3 (March, 1979) 336

[19] Cunningham, MacDonald, and Gant 818

[20] Cunningham, MacDonald, and Gant 819

[21] Cunningham, MacDonald, and Gant 818

Chapter III

[1] Sheldon B. Korones, High Risk Newborn Infants: The Basis for Intensive Nursing Care (St. Louis: The C.V. Mosby Co., 1986) 22

[2] Korones 22

RESOURCES

<u>Organizations</u>
Check your phone book for local addresses and phone numbers

American Diabetes Association
 1660 Duke St.
 Alexandria, VA 22314
 1-800-232-3472
  Information re: Diabetes, diabetes and pregnancy, gestational diabetes.

American Heart Association
 7272 Greenville Ave.
 Dallas, TX 75231-4596
 1-800-242-1793
  Information re: hypertension, pregnancy-induced hypertension, congenital heart defects, and more.

The Compassionate Friends
 P.O. Box 3696
 Oak Brook, IL 60522-3696
 (708) 990-0010
  Support groups, support services, grief counseling for those who have experienced miscarriage or death of infant.

International Childbirth Education Association
 P.O. Box 20048
 Minneapolis, MN 55420-0048
 (612) 854-8660
  Information and classes re: childbirth, breast-feeding, parenting.

National Organization of Mothers of Twins Clubs, Inc.
 P.O. Box 23188
 Albuquerque, NM 87192-1188
 (505) 275-0955
  Support group for mothers of twins. Fathers invited. Quarterly newsletter. Monthly meetings with speakers. Fathers' night. Parties.

Organizations

Resolve, Inc.
　　1310 Broadway
　　Somerville, MA 02144-1731
　　(617) 623-0744

Sidelines
　　2805 Park Place
　　Laguna Beach, CA 92651
　　(714) 497-2265
　　　　National network of local support groups for women
　　　　experiencing complicated pregnancies. Newsletter, phone
　　　　contacts, peer counselors. Call the national office for
　　　　information about the support group closest to you.

Triplet Connection
　　P.O. Box 99571
　　Stockton, CA 95209
　　(209) 474-0885
　　　　National network of information and support groups for
　　　　families of triplets, quads, and quints. Informational
　　　　packets sent to expectant parents of multiples. Quarterly
　　　　national newsletter. Database of information about
　　　　multiples. Expert scientific counsel.

Books

Parenting Your Premature Baby
>   by Janice Jason, M.D. and Antonia Van Der Meer
>   Holt & Co., New York, 1989

Pregnancy Bedrest: A Guidebook for the Pregnant Woman and Her Family.
>   by Susan H. Johnston and Deborah A. Kraut
>   Holt & Co., New York, 1990

The Premature Baby Book
>   by Helen Harrison
>   St. Martin's Press, 1983

When Pregnancy Isn't Perfect
>   by Laurie A. Rich
>   Dutton, Penguin Books, 1991.

INDEX

ORDER FORM

Please send a copy of:

BEDREST BEFORE BABY:
WHAT'S A MOTHER TO DO?
A Survival Handbook for High Risk Moms

to:

Name:_____

Address:_____

_____

Zip Code:_____

Phone #:(___)_____

BEDREST BEFORE BABY	$ 12.95
Sales tax (Maryland addresses only: $.65)	___.___
Shipping - surface: $1.50 (allow 3 - 4 weeks for delivery)	___.___
Air mail: $3.00	___.___
Total	$___.___

Make checks payable to: Mustard Seed Publications

Mail to: 9904 Gunforge Road
Suite 925
Perry Hall, MD 21128-9518